Interventional Pulmonology and Pulmonary Hypertension - Updates on Specific Topics

Edited by Theodoros Aslanidis

Published in London, United Kingdom

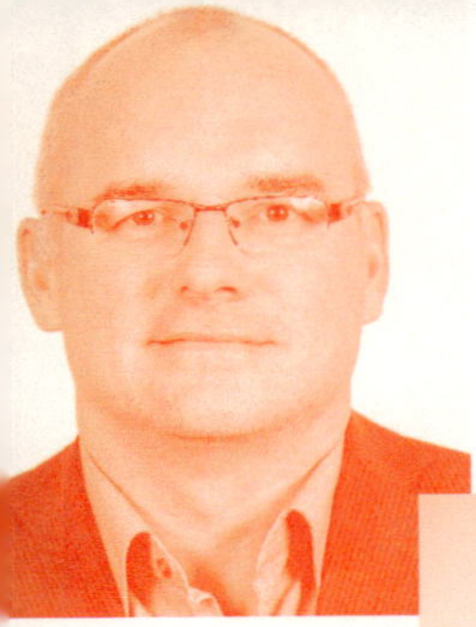
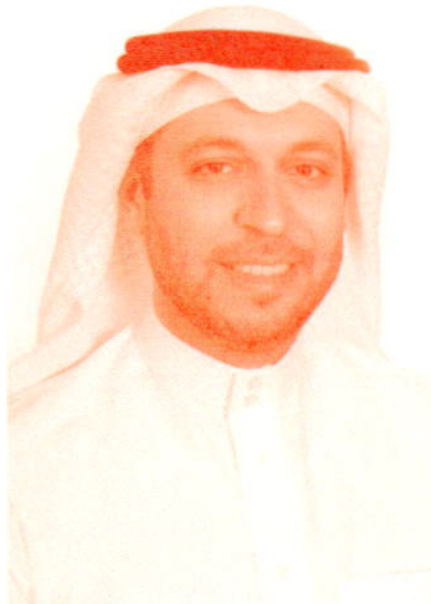
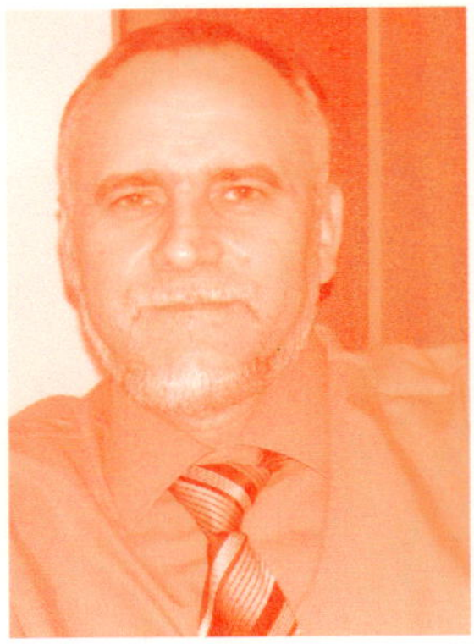
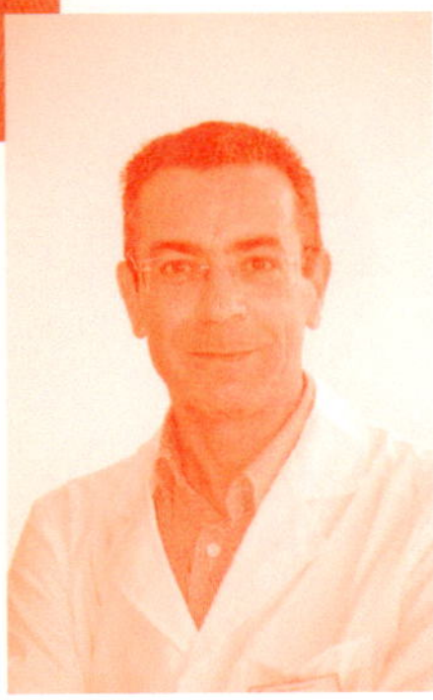
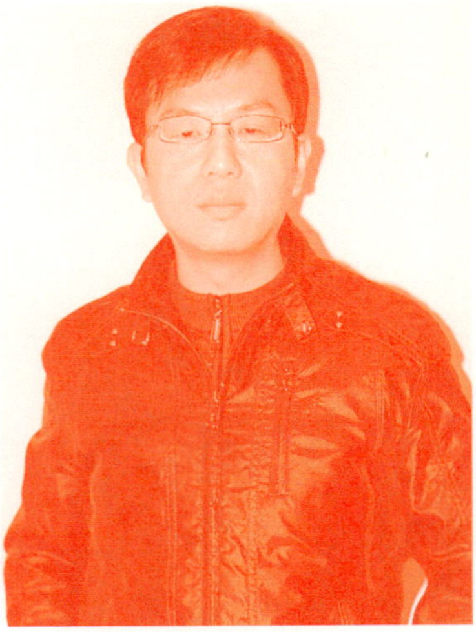
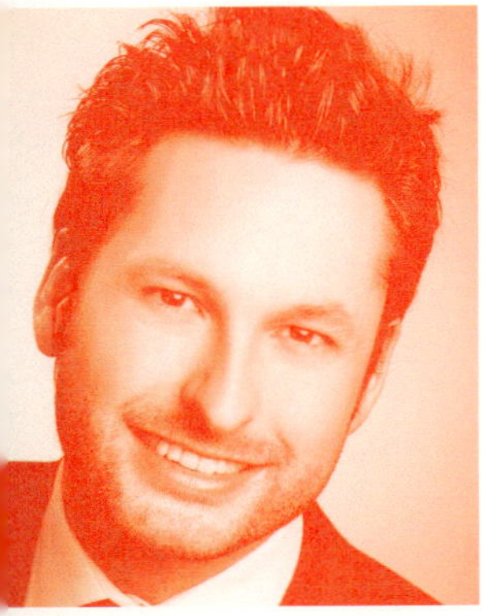
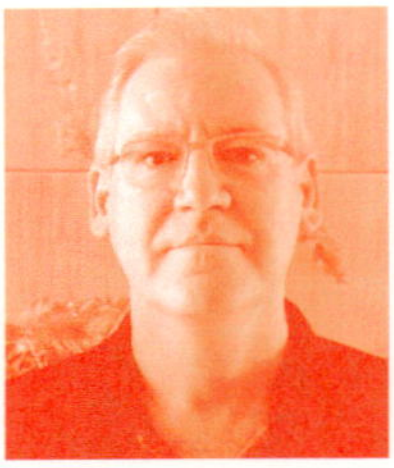

IntechOpen

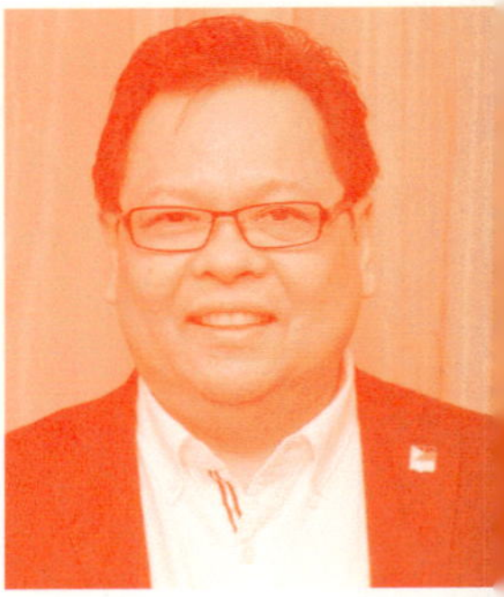
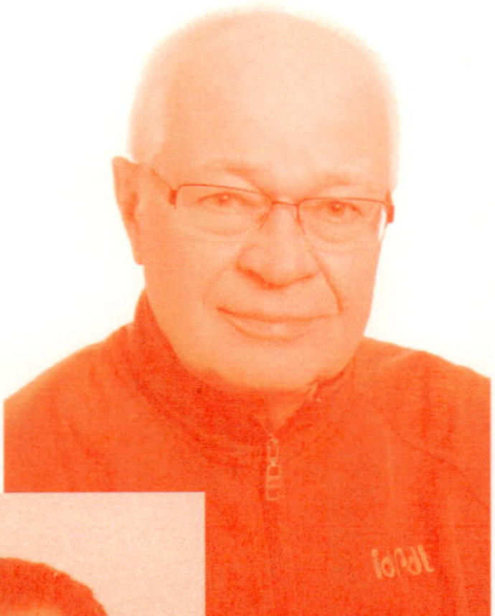
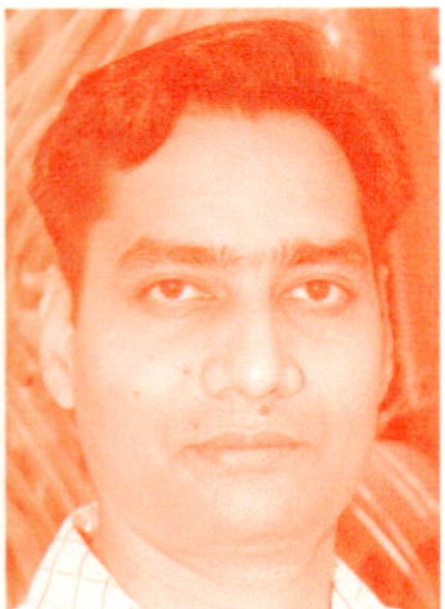
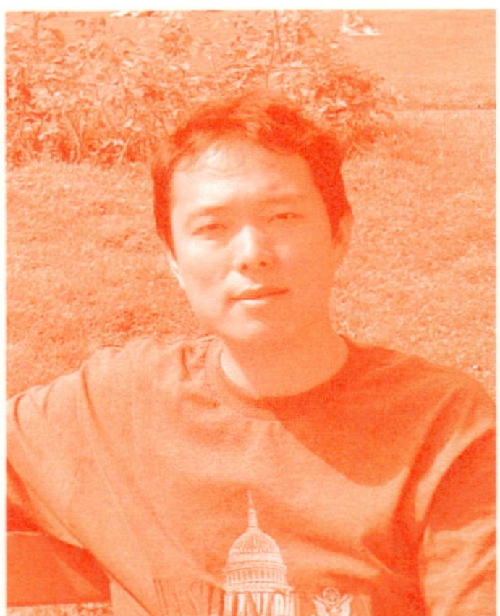
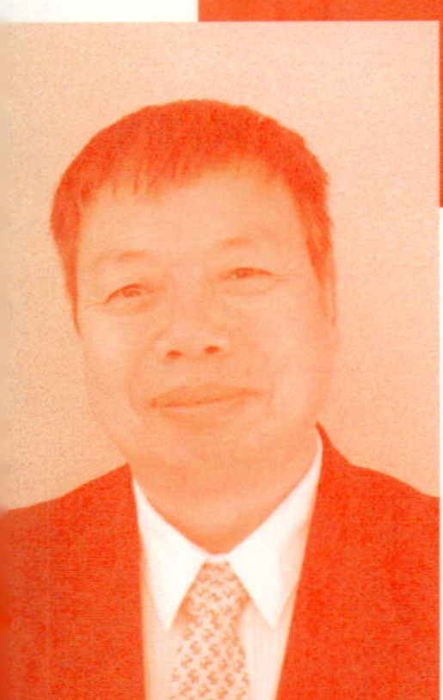
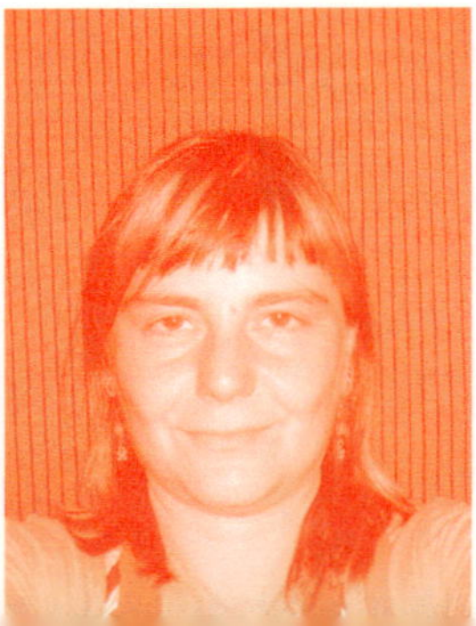

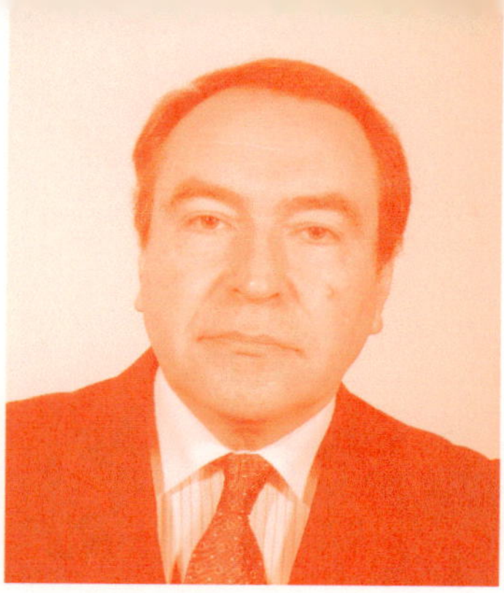

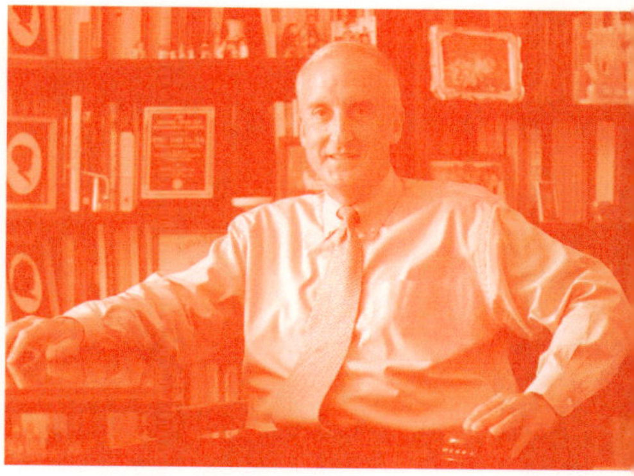

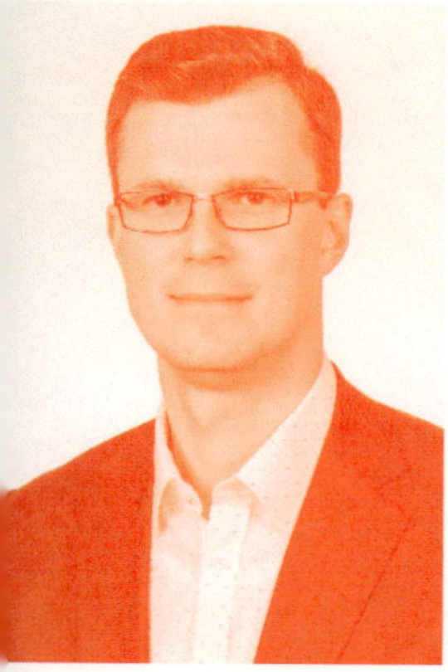

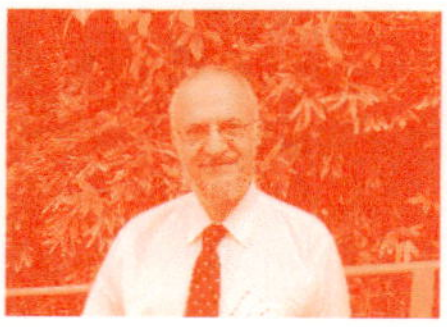

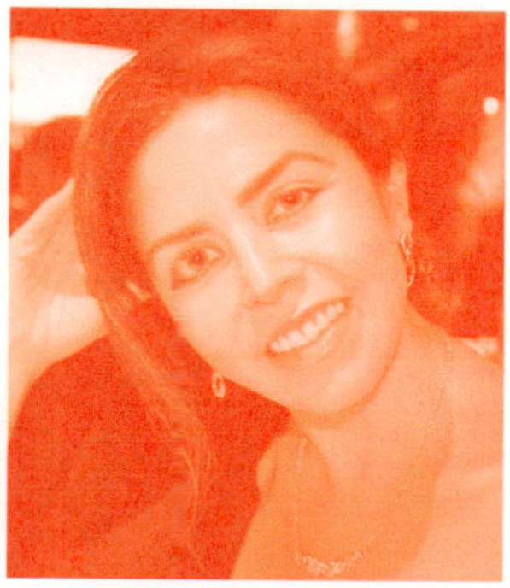

Supporting open minds since 2005

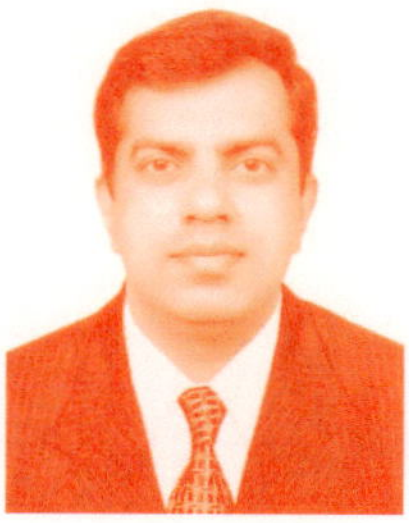

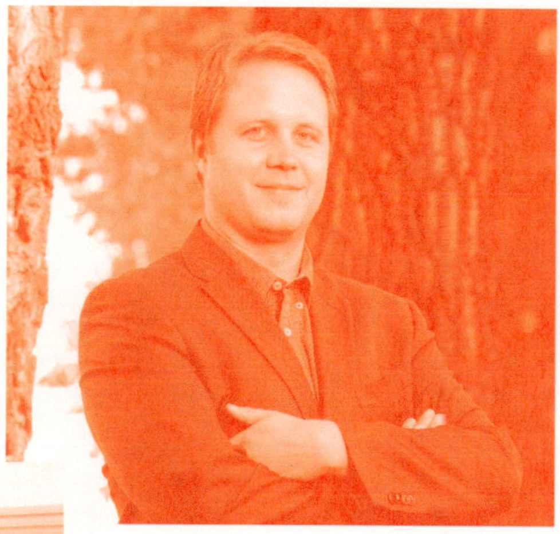

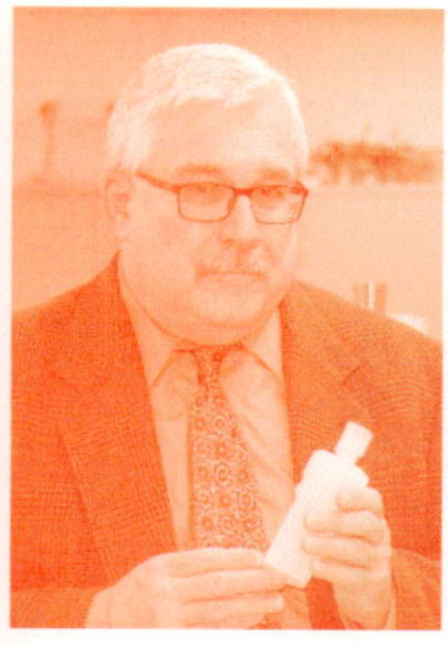

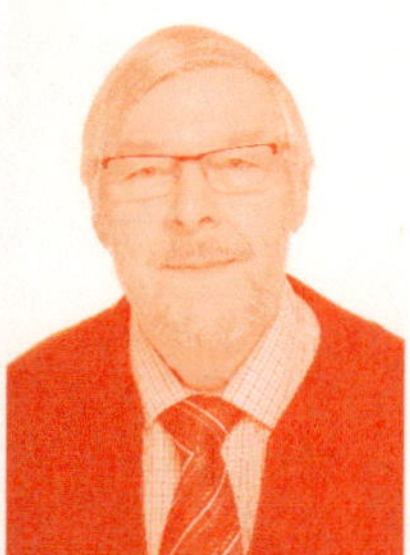

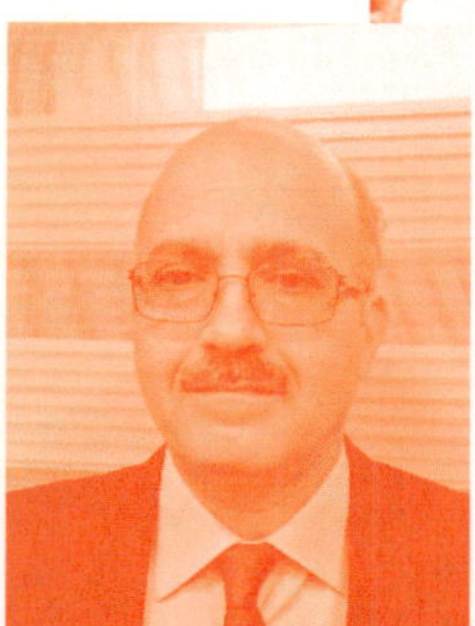

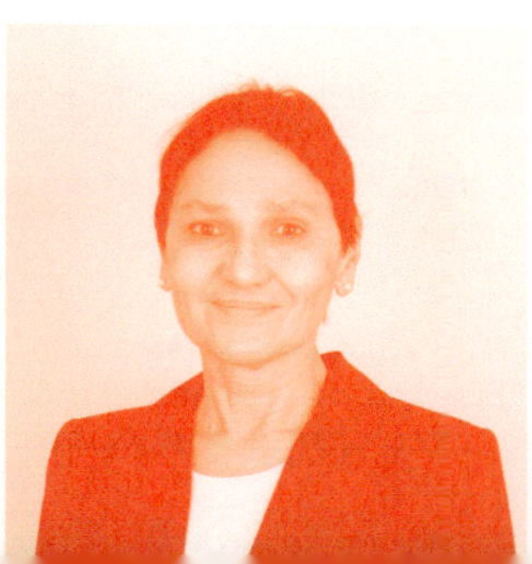

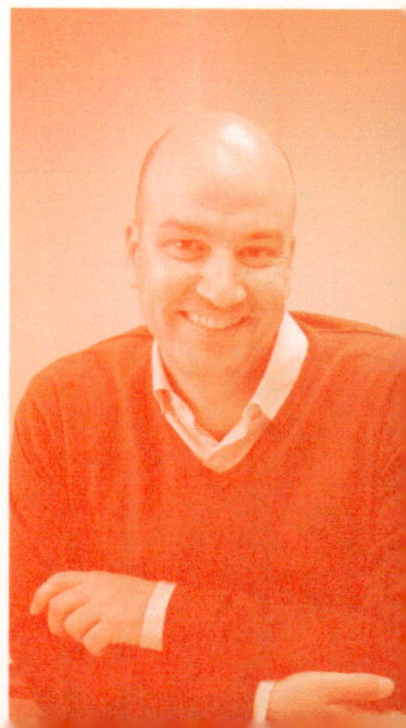

Interventional Pulmonology and Pulmonary Hypertension - Updates on Specific Topics
http://dx.doi.org/10.5772/intechopen.78454
Edited by Theodoros Aslanidis

Contributors
Yousef Shweihat, Shantanu Singh, Sachin Kumar, Petr Kotlyarov, Stevan Tofovic, Edwin Jackson, Theodoros Aslanidis, Vitalie Faoro, Kevin Forton

First published in London, United Kingdom, 2020 by IntechOpen
IntechOpen is the global imprint of INTECHOPEN LIMITED, registered in England and Wales, registration number: 11086078, 7th floor, 10 Lower Thames Street, London, EC3R 6AF, United Kingdom
Printed in Croatia

British Library Cataloguing-in-Publication Data
A catalogue record for this book is available from the British Library

Additional hard and PDF copies can be obtained from orders@intechopen.com

Interventional Pulmonology and Pulmonary Hypertension - Updates on Specific Topics
Edited by Theodoros Aslanidis
p. cm.
Print ISBN 978-1-78984-041-4
Online ISBN 978-1-78984-042-1
eBook (PDF) ISBN 978-1-83880-418-3

For EU product safety concerns:
IN TECH d.o.o., Prolaz Marije Krucifikse Kozulić 3, 51000 Rijeka, Croatia, info@intechopen.com or visit our website at intechopen.com.

Meet the editor

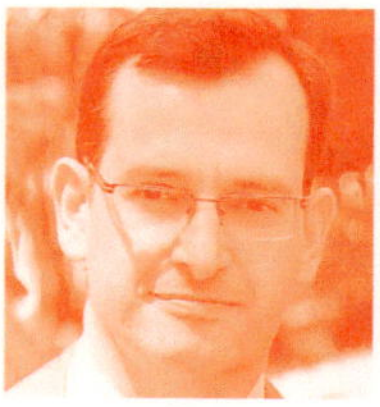

Dr. Theodoros Aslanidis received his Doctor of Medicine degree from the Medical University, Plovdiv, Bulgaria, and his PhD degree from the Aristotle Medical University of Thessaloniki, Greece. He served in the Hellenic Army Force as a medical doctor and then worked as a rural physician at the Outhealth Centre, Iraklia, and Serres' General Hospital, Greece. He completed his residency in anesthesiology at "Hippokratio" General Hospital, with a subspecialty in critical care training at the AHEPA University Hospital and a postgraduate program in prehospital emergency medicine from the National Centre of Emergency Care, where he served as an EMS physician and emergency communication center medic. Currently, he is working as a consultant-researcher at the intensive care unit of St. Paul General Hospital, Thessaloniki, Greece. He serves as an editor for multiple medical journals. His research interests are medical writing, data analysis, emergency critical care, and neuromonitoring.

Contents

Preface

Pulmonary medicine obviously continues to be a discipline that is attracting bright, dedicated, and sincerely adventurous individuals, a discipline that is rapidly evolving and changing. Though asthma and chronic obstructive pulmonary disease still claim the role of "kings" in respiratory medicine, huge progress is being made also in other areas.

Today, we live in an era of transition for pulmonologists, prompting John Hansen-Flaschen, Professor of Medicine at the University of Pennsylvania, to call them "spironauts": scientists with a wider role both in critical care and sleep medicine.

Within this frame, this book, published by IntechOpen, focuses on interesting aspects of pulmonary medicine. The first section of the book is dedicated to interventional pulmonology, and includes updates on bronchial thermoplasty, virtual bronchoscopy, and endobronchial ultrasound. The second section highlights special aspects of pulmonary circulation and pulmonary hypertension. Throughout the book, the authors offer us not only a "vigorous" review of the current literature but also a research path to further advancement.

Dr. Theodoros Aslanidis
Intensive Care Unit,
St. Paul General Hospital,
Thessaloniki, Greece

Section 1

Introduction

Chapter 1

Introductory Chapter: Whole Lung Lavage for Pulmonary Alveolar Proteinosis—The Challenges Remain

Theodoros Aslanidis

1. Pulmonary alveolar proteinosis

Since its first description in 1958 by Samuel H. Rosen et al., understanding pulmonary alveolar proteinosis (PAP) (or pulmonary alveolar lipoproteinosis or pulmonary alveolar phospholipidosis) has made a tremendous advance [1].

Today, PAP remains a rare lung disease. Prevalence ranges from 3.7 to 40 cases per million, depending on the country, and the incidence has been estimated to be 0.2 cases per million. The main pathological mechanism behind the disease is the accumulation of lipoproteinaceous material in the alveoli due to dysfunctional clearance by alveolar macrophages or type II epithelial cells. There are three clinically distinct forms: (1) congenital, caused by mutations in the CSF2RA gene on chromosome Xp22.33 or impaired CSF2RB expression. The result is a dysfunctional α or β granulocyte-macrophage colony-stimulating factor (GM-CSF) receptor subunit. (2) Secondary pulmonary alveolar proteinosis develops in association with conditions involving functional impairment or reduced numbers of alveolar macrophages (hematologic cancers, pharmacologic immunosuppression, inhalation of inorganic dust or toxic fumes, and certain infections). (3) Finally, autoimmune PAP is initiated by immunoglobulin (Ig)-G anti-granulocyte-macrophage colony-stimulating factor (anti-GM-CSF) antibodies, which decrease functional alveolar macrophages [2].

Clinical presentation of PAP varies: dyspnea, cough, hemoptysis, fever, and chest pain appear in a different range, while signs of chronic respiratory failure (cyanosis, clubbing, inspiratory crackles) can be found in clinical examination.

Diagnosis demands appropriate serological, radiological, and bronchoscopic evaluation and opting out other interstitial lung diseases [3].

2. Therapeutic options

Unfortunately, apart from the conditions in which etiological therapy is available, therapeutic options remain limited. Supplementation of exogenous granulocyte-macrophage colony-stimulating factor (GM-CSF) or strategies aimed at reducing the levels of the autoantibodies, like plasmapheresis or rituximab—a monoclonal antibody directed against the CD20 antigen of B-lymphocytes and ameliorates PAP by decreasing anti-GM-CSF antibody concentration—are promising approaches. Other options like stem cell or lung transplantation have more limited use.

On the other hand, whole lung lavage (WLL) is the standard first-line therapy [4]. Theoretic concept behind WLL is simple. Clinical and physiological improvement is caused by the removal of lipoproteinaceous material and anti-GM-CSF antibodies from the alveolar space. Additional immunological effects on the effector cells (e.g., alveolar macrophages or type II epithelial cells) may also be included.

3. Whole lung lavage: the challenges

Due to the rarity of the disease, there are no guidelines regarding technical details about WLL. Usually, a dedicated team, which includes experienced anesthesia and respiratory nurses, anesthesiologist, respiratory physiotherapist, and a pulmonologist experienced in interventional pulmonology, is needed to perform the procedure [5].

Indications for WLL also vary. In general, dyspnea-induced limitation of daily activities is the rule, although decline in SpO_2 (>70% in room air), radiographic worsening, decline in DLCO or FVC, and other symptoms have also been used [6].

Thus, timing between diagnosis of PAP and WLL varies from 2 months to 17 years, although most of the patients need WLL within a year from diagnosis [5]. Time of repeating WLL depends on patient's condition [2]. Available literature reports an interval between 15 months and 3 years [7, 8]. Three (3) weeks interval between right and left lung WLL is considered safe and long enough for clinical improvement to arise [6]. However, bilateral WLL has also been performed without any problems [9].

Usually, the procedure is performed first in the most severely affected lung. Imaging techniques such as perfusion/ventilation scan can help in the final selection. Patient is positioned usually supine, although multiple positions, like lateral decubitus, Trendelenburg, and prone, have also been reported [10].

The procedure is carried out under general anesthesia. The preferred technique is total intravenous anesthesia, while volatile anesthetics has been used in cases of bronchospasm. After preoxygenation, a left double-lumen endotracheal tube (DLT) with minimum size 26 Fr is used for intubation and lung isolation. Right DLT is avoided due to risk of right upper lobe orifice block [6]. Recently, there also reports—still rare—of noninvasive ventilation (NIV) as alternative to intubation with DLT [11]. The same is valid also for anesthesia, as reports are published for WLL during local anesthesia and the use of fiber-optic bronchoscope [12].

Hypoxemia is common during WLL. Several strategies are suggested in order to cope with the problem: positive end-expiratory pressure (PEEP) application, manual ventilation of partially fluid-filled lung, intermittent double-lung ventilation, concomitant use of inhaled nitric oxide, ipsilateral occlusion of pulmonary artery of the non-ventilated lung via pulmonary artery catheter, hyperbaric oxygen therapy, and parallel use of veno-venous extracorporeal membrane oxygenation (ECMO) [6, 10, 13–16]. No guideline or data exist for the use of one method over the others.

In most of the literature warmed (to 37°C) NaCl 0.9% is reported as lung fluid. The total volume needed ranges from 30 to 50 liters [6]. The fluid can flow by gravitational force in 500–1000 ml or FRC equivalent volume aliquots for 10–30 cycles. The maximum pressure allowed should be below the sealing pressure of the ventilated lung (between 30 and 50 cm). In case of fiber-optic bronchoscopic lavage under local anesthesia, 50 ml aliquots are used [12].

The mechanism of protein transfer from the surfactant and blood into the lavage fluid during WLL has not been sufficiently studied. A recent report suggests a mathematical model—expressed with several differential equations—based on diffusion for the transfer of most of the substances. However, there are still components of the alveolar proteinaceous material—mainly with low molecular weight—which do not follow the suggested model [17].

Chest percussion with a wraparound vest or manual percussion by a physiotherapist is applied for 3–5 minutes, in order to increase clearance of proteinaceous material. This can be performed throughout the procedure (from installation to removal of the fluid). Till now, there is no comparative study for the method of percussion; still, some authors claim that mechanical percussion with vest is best tolerated [10].

Intraoperative monitoring varies, yet it generally includes invasive arterial blood pressure for serial arterial blood gases examination. Recently, lung ultrasound has been also suggested as a promising method of monitoring the amount of saline used for lavage and pick-up complications like pleural effusion [18].

In the immediate post-procedure phase, diuretics can help clearing fluid from the lung [8], while follow-up is usually performed via chest X-ray or computer tomography imaging [6].

Complication rate ranges from 0.8% for pneumothorax to 18% for transient fever; other complications are hypoxemia, pleural effusion, pneumonia, wheezing, etc. [6].

Long-term efficiency of the procedure is generally good, though available literature is limited.

4. Conclusion: time for a consensus?

Almost 70 years after its first application and despite the lack of an alternative option, WLL performance and efficiency continues to rely mostly on local expertise and experience. Yet, as the available database knowledge is increasing (especially after 1990) and the indication for WLL include more and more conditions (i.e., pneumoconiosis, silicosis, lipoid pneumonia), it may be the time for a guideline or for a minimum consensus upon to improve future procedure's safety and efficiency and facilitate everyday clinical decision-making.

Conflict of interests

The author has no conflict of interest.

Author details

Theodoros Aslanidis
Intensive Care Unit, St. Paul General Hospital, Thessaloniki, Greece

*Address all correspondence to: thaslan@hotmail.com

References

[1] Rosen SH, Castleman B, Liebow AA. Pulmonary alveolar proteinosis. The New England Journal of Medicine. 1958;**258**(23):1123-1142

[2] Borie R, Danel C, Debray MP, Taille C, Dombret MC, Aubier M, et al. Pulmonary alveolar proteinosis. European Respiratory Review. 2011;**20**(120):98-107

[3] Campo I, Mariani F, Rodi G, Paracchini E, Tsana E, Piloni D, et al. Assessment and management of pulmonary alveolar proteinosis in a reference center. Orphanet Journal of Rare Diseases. 2013;**8**:40

[4] Suzuki T, Trapnell BC. Pulmonary alveolar proteinosis syndrome. Clinics in Chest Medicine. 2016;**37**(3):431-440

[5] Gay P, Wallaert B, Nowak S, Yserbyt J, Anevlavis S, Hermant C, et al. Efficacy of whole-lung lavage in pulmonary alveolar proteinosis: A multicenter international study of GELF. Respiration. 2017;**93**:198-120

[6] Campo I, Luisetti M, Griese M, et al. Whole lung lavage therapy for pulmonary alveolar proteinosis: A global survey of current practices and procedures. Orphanet Journal of Rare Diseases. 2016;**11**:115

[7] Seymour JF, Presneill JJ. Pulmonary alveolar proteinosis: Progress in the first 44 years. American Journal of Respiratory and Critical Care Medicine. 2002;**166**:215-235

[8] Beccaria M, Luisetti M, Rodi G, et al. Long-term durable benefit after whole lung lavage in pulmonary alveolar proteinosis. The European Respiratory Journal. 2004;**23**:526-531

[9] Silva A, Moreto A, Pinho C, et al. Bilateral whole lung lavage in pulmonary alveolar proteinosis—A retrospective study. Revista Portuguesa de Pneumologia. 2014;**20**:254-259

[10] Awab A, Khan MS, Youness HA. Whole lung lavage-technical details, challenges and management of complications. Journal of Thoracic Disease. 2017;**9**(6):1697-1706

[11] Skoczynski S, Wyskida K, Rzepka-Wrona P, et al. Novel method of noninvasive ventilation supported therapeutic lavage in pulmonary alveolar proteinosis proves to relieve dyspnea, normalize pulmonary function test results and recover exercise capacity: A short communication. Journal of Thoracic Disease. 2018;**10**(4):2467-2473

[12] Cheng S, Chang HI, Lau HP, Lee LN, Yang PC. Treatment by bronchofiberscopic lobar lavage: Pulmonary alveolar proteinosis. Chest. 2002;**122**:1480-1485

[13] Rebelo H, Guedes L, Veiga D, Fiuza A, Abelha F. Anaesthetic, procedure and complication management serial lung lavagein an obese patient with alveolar proteinosis: A case report. Revista Brasileira de Anestesiologia. 2012;**62**(6):869-877

[14] Ahmed R, Iqbal M, Kashef SH, Almomatten MI. Whole lung lavage with intermittent double lung ventilation. A modified technique for managing pulmonary alveolar proteinosis. Saudi Medical Journal. 2005;**26**(1):139141

[15] Moutafis M, Dalibon N, Colchen A, Fischler M. Improving oxygenation during bronchopulmonary lavage using nitric oxide inhalation and almitrine infusion. Anesthesia and Analgesia. 1999;**89**(2):302

[16] Nadeau MJ, Côté D, Bussières JS. The combination of inhaled nitric oxide

and pulmonary artery balloon inflation improves oxygenation during whole-lung lavage. Anesthesia and Analgesia. 2004;**99**(3):676-679

[17] Akasaka K, Tanaka T, Maruyama T, Kitamura N, Hashimoto A, Ito Y, et al. A mathematical model to predict protein wash out kinetics during whole-lung lavage in autoimmune pulmonary alveolar proteinosis. American Journal of Physiology. Lung Cellular and Molecular Physiology. 2015;**308**:L105-L117. (First published November 14, 2014. DOI: 10.1152/ajplung.00239.2014

[18] Ramachandran P, Chaudhury A, Devaraj U, Maheshwari KU, D'Souza G. Monitoring whole-lung lavage using lung ultrasound: The changing phases of the lung. Lung India. 2018;**35**:350-353

Section 2

Interventional Pulmonology

Chapter 2

EUS-B for the Interventional Pulmonologist Using the EBUS Scope in the Esophagus

Yousef R. Shweihat and Shantanu Singh

Abstract

This chapter aims at introducing the interested Pulmonologist/Interventional Pulmonologist to the esophageal ultrasound. In this chapter, we give short descriptions of some technical aspects of the endobronchial ultrasound (EBUS) scope and explain in detail why we believe the EBUS scope is well suited to be an esophageal scope in the hands of the trained pulmonologist. The chapter then explains indications and benefits of this procedure that we consider central to the practice of chest physicians. We also describe in steps how to reach each lymph node station using the EBUS scope as a EUS scope (EUS-B) from our own experience. Procedure-related complications and contraindications are also described.

Keywords: esophageal ultrasound, endobronchial ultrasound, lymph node stations

1. Introduction

Interventional pulmonary has witnessed substantial growth in the past few years. A major factor in the growth has been the advent of endobronchial ultrasound (EBUS) as a staging modality for lung cancer and as a diagnostic tool for diseases with mediastinal involvement. The development of EBUS was preceded by esophageal ultrasound (EUS), and the literatures on both techniques have grown in parallel. More recently, the efficacy and utility of an esophageal approach using the EBUS scope (EUS-B) has been described to access nodes and masses accessible during a single sedation to more accurately diagnose and stage disease either via tracheal or esophageal route. Here, we describe relevant anatomy, procedural techniques, indications, contraindications, and complications for EUS-B.

2. Technical aspects

2.1 EBUS bronchoscope

EBUS can refer to two distinct types of probes/scopes. Radial probe EBUS is the first type, and was commercially available in 1992. It increased the yield of transbronchial needle aspiration of mediastinal lymph nodes and is currently used mainly to biopsy peripheral nodules or examines the different central airways diseases. The second type is the convex/curvilinear probe EBUS bronchoscope. It was introduced in 2002 and commercialized around 2004. In this chapter, our discussion is limited to the most widely available curvilinear scope manufactured by multiple companies (Olympus, Fuji, and Pentax) with minimal differences in characteristics. The differences between scopes are beyond the scope of this text. The reader is encouraged to be familiar with the specifications of the scopes and their relative US processors available at his/her institution. Some features are worth mentioning though which are big difference between the EBUS and conventional EUS scopes. The working tube of about 60 cm is much shorter than the EUS. The largest intubating diameter at the tip of the EBUS scopes ranges from 6.7 to 7.4 mm. The remainder of the insertion tubes has a diameter of 6.3–6.4 mm. The working channel diameter is from 2.0 to 2.2 mm. The ultrasonic transducer is situated at the tip of the bronchoscope just distal to the video camera, light source, and the working channel aperture. It emits ultrasonic waves that range from 5 to 12 MHz, and this depends on the ultrasound processor used and settings selected. The ultrasonic scanning range obtained via these scopes is triangular in shape and yields a 60–75° view parallel to the insertion tube. The tissue depth of ultrasonic views and focusing capabilities can be altered and varies according to the ultrasound processor used. Multiple manufacturers offer single-use aspiration needles available in 19G, 21G, and 22G with excellent puncture capability under ultrasonic view. The design improves visibility on ultrasound images to enable a precise puncture. After loading and securing the needle in the working channel, the needle extends out of the channel and intersects with the ultrasonic view enabling the endoscopist to control the depth and location of needle insertion into the lymph node in a real time fashion.

2.2 Why the EBUS scope, not the EUS scope?

The EBUS scope is different in many ways from its counterpart used in the GI tract. **First**, the diameter is almost half of any available ultrasound endoscope. In our opinion, this makes the bronchoscope more comfortable for the patient, and reduces sedation requirement. **Second**, the control part of the bronchoscope has fewer controllers making it easier for the pulmonologist to handle. It is a design that they are used to and comfortable using with no need for extra training to be able to handle it. This in our opinion shortens the learning curve. **Third**, it enables the thoracic physician to completely evaluate the mediastinum in one session using one piece of equipment. This minimizes the costs of additional equipment and need for additional procedure without compromising on patient management. **Fourth**, the EBUS scope is shorter than the EUS scope, thus enhancing maneuverability. This shorter length is well suited for sampling thoracic and mediastinal structures. Sampling of the pancreas or abdominal lymph nodes is out of the scope and expertise of most thoracic physicians. Added length of the EUS scope does not offer additional advantage to a practicing pulmonologist.

3. Indications

One of the major advances in the treatment of lung cancer is the advent of non-surgical pathologic staging using EBUS. The combination of EBUS and EUS for sampling of mediastinal nodes allows near complete staging of the mediastinum [1–3], which is equivalent, if not superior to mediastinoscopy in experienced hands [4, 5]. Multiple studies showed the EBUS scope efficacious in serving the EUS scope role (EUS-B) [6, 7]. The added benefit of the esophageal access in staging lung cancer comes from its ability to reach and locate lymph nodal stations that are impossible to reach via the airways such as stations 3p, and paraesophageal lymph nodal

Lymph node station	EBUS	EUS-B
1	+	–
2R	+	+
2L	+	+
3a	–	–
3p	–	+
4R	+	–
4L	+	+
5	–	+
6	–	*
7	+	+
8 R,L	–	+
9 R,L	–	+
10–12 R,L	+	–

**reported using EUS but not EUS-B.*

Table 1.
Lymph nodes accessible by EBUS vs. EUS-B.

Indications for EUS-B
Lung cancer staging, stations 3p, 8, 9, 5, and 4L and 7
Paraesophageal abnormalities not accessible via the airways
Mediastinal masses that can be approached through airway and esophagus, esophagus is preferred for patient comfort
Sampling mediastinal lymphadenopathy of any etiology
Mediastinal pathology in critically ill or intubated patients
Sampling and drainage of mediastinal cysts
Bleeding diathesis (see text)

Table 2.
Indications for EUS-B.

stations 8 and 9 (see **Table 1** for lymph node stations accessible by EBUS and EUS). Given the literature on combined EBUS and EUS, it can be argued that EBUS and EUS-B should be performed at the same time for all patients with suspected lung cancer at institutions where rapid on-site cytologic evaluation is not available. This approach is recommended by the European Society of Gastrointestinal Endoscopy (ESGE) and European Respiratory Society (ERS) guidelines [8]. The utility of EBUS and EUS-B is not limited to staging or diagnosis of lung cancer. The EBUS has well documented advantages in diagnosing mediastinal lymphoma [9–11], sarcoidosis [12–14], tuberculosis [15, 16], pulmonary parenchymal masses [17, 18], and metastatic disease to the mediastinum [19], among others including infections [9, 20]. EUS-B has the same ability to investigate the mediastinum when such conditions are suspected, since the utility of EUS is well documented in such disease states [21, 22]. In addition, instances where a mediastinal mass or lymphadenopathy is paraesophageal and paratracheal, the esophageal approach might be preferred, especially when there is difficulty to access the airway due to patient intolerance or if accessing the airway predisposes increase risk to hypoxemic, intubated, and critically ill patients [23]. The indications for EUS-B are summarized in **Table 2**.

4. Anesthesia

EBUS bronchoscopy is carried out under either conscious sedation or general anesthesia with laryngeal mask airway (LMA) or intubation. EUS/B can be performed in the same setting under general anesthesia or conscious sedation. Patient tolerance seems to be adequate when conscious sedation is used [24]. Multiple drug regimens are available for conscious sedation. We do not recommend one regimen over the other. Local expertise, hospital policies, availability of an anesthesia team, and costs govern the types of sedatives and techniques used. Institutional protocols should be developed and followed to ensure safety of procedures. Even when LMA is used, EUS-B can still be performed in the same setting as described below. This is one benefit of EUS-B over conventional EUS. It is important to mention in this setting that endotracheal intubation is not prohibitive of performing EUS-B and is actually an indication as mentioned earlier. In the intubated and/or the critically ill patient, EUS-B allows us the easiest and sometimes the only access to mediastinal pathology. It is our experience that this approach does not require more sedation than required for mechanical ventilation.

5. Insertion techniques for EUS-B

It is necessary to intubate the oral cavity (as opposed to the nares) when using the EBUS scope. A "bite block" (in cases of intubation, in ICU and conscious sedation) should be used to protect the scope from potential damage from a bite if LMA is not used. An added oropharyngeal airway, such as the Williams airway, can facilitate passage of the scope into the supraglottic/posterior pharyngeal space and offer further protection to scope under conscious sedation.

When conscious sedation or endotracheal (ET) tube is used and once in the posterior pharyngeal space, the scope can be advanced into the esophagus using two basic techniques. The first "blind" technique involves holding the scope with the ultrasound transducer facing the posterior pharynx. Patient is instructed to swallow after instillation of topical lidocaine or saline. Once the patient starts swallowing, the

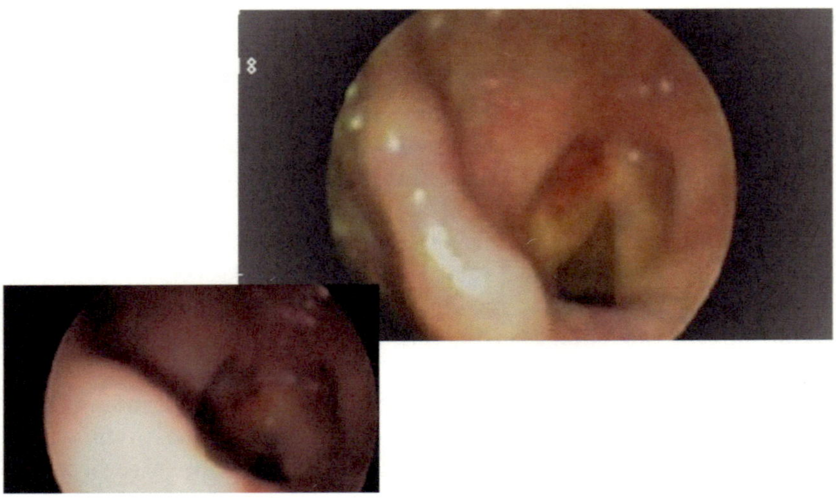

Figure 1.
After bypassing the epiglottis, to enter the esophagus, the scope needs to be placed behind the left arytenoid. Vision will cease after that point and US vision should be used to assist locating the probe position in the esophagus. Note: gentle pressure with some corkscrew or alternating mild upward and downward movements on the scope lever will assist in entering the esophagus.

scope can be advanced with gentle pressure, allowing the peristaltic wave to carry it. Rapid minor alternating flexion and release of the scope using the control lever can aid passage of the scope into the esophagus. If the blind technique fails, the scope can be passed under direct visualization. The scope can be inserted with the transducer (and visual field) facing anteriorly. Once in the posterior pharynx, the tip can be retroflexed and the larynx visualized. The tip of the scope can then be passed posterior to the arytenoids and to left with gentle pressure, see **Figure 1**. If resistance is faced, the scope can be withdrawn and another attempt on the right side or midline can be tried. It is important not to use excessive pressure if the scope does not pass easily. A gentle corkscrew maneuver with gentle advancement is all that is required.

The use of the LMA is prohibitive of using the conventional EUS scope but not the EUS-B. The LMA inherently obstructs the esophageal opening. Once the EBUS scope is at the level of the larynx, the tip is pointed and scope placed behind the left arytenoid. An assistant is asked to perform a jaw thrust maneuver that will elevate the laryngeal structures and give enough space for the small EBUS scope to be gently passed into the esophagus. Once in the esophagus, the jaw thrust can be stopped and procedure is continued. In our experience, with over 500 EUS-B procedures, we have not experienced failure or a complication passing the scope into the esophagus using any of these techniques.

6. Anatomic landmarks and organs studied

In contrast to EBUS in the airways, EUS-B relies entirely upon ultrasonic images for localization; the esophagus has no internal landmarks for nodal mapping. Because of this, lymph node stations are identified and numbered based upon their relationships with other structures "seen" ultrasonographically through esophageal wall. In addition, interpersonal variability exists between patients, and large mediastinal tumors or abnormalities can alter the normal anatomy and displace or compress the esophagus or other structures, thus altering the ultrasonic views and anatomic relations. A computerized tomographic scan is almost invariably available. It is advised that the endoscopist carefully review patient anatomy prior to and during the procedure to avoid sampling normal structures.

The mediastinal structures that can be normally seen and examined on EUS-B are:

1. Cardiac structures: left atrium, left ventricle, aortic valve, mitral valve, pericardium

2. Thoracic aorta: descending, arch, root

3. Pulmonary vessels: left pulmonary artery, right pulmonary artery

4. Vertebral bodies

5. Mediastinal pleura and pleural effusion if large enough

6. Mediastinal lymph nodes

7. Liver

During the initial training for EUS, it is important to define a point of reference that the endoscopist can refer to during the procedure. In our practice, we first identify the left atrium as a point of reference. The scope is advanced into

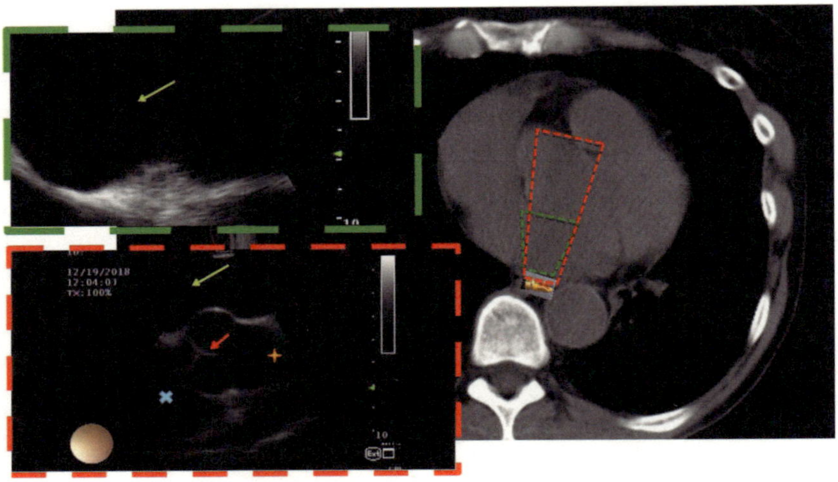

Figure 2.
At 3–4 cm depth (dashed green), the left atrium (green arrow) can be seen looking anteriorly. Increasing the depth to 5–7 cm and slight rotation can identify the aortic valve (red arrow), root (orange star), and outflow tract from left ventricle (blue x).

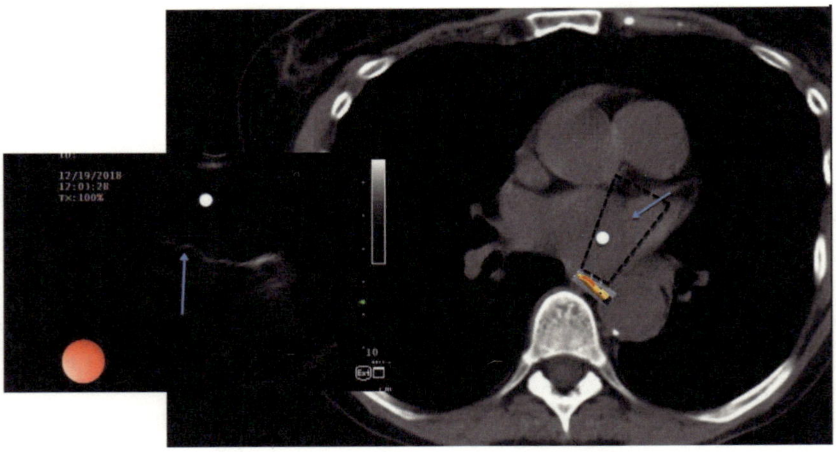

Figure 3.
Moving distally with slight rotation to left and increased depth can show the mitral valve (blue arrow) under the LA (white circle).

the esophagus with the ultrasound transducer facing anteriorly until the atrium can be identified. The atrium is easily identified due to its shape, its pulsating nature, and great variability in size (compared to the great vessels) with contractions (**Figure 2**, also see Video at https://mts.intechopen.com/download/index/process/324/authkey/bb9c02ba5640a4d21d4511e0a79f3621). A thin paper-like echogenic structure can usually be observed moving inside of this anechoic sac (of blood), this is the mitral valve (**Figure 3**, also see Video at https://mts.intechopen.com/download/index/process/324/authkey/bb9c02ba5640a4d21d4511e0a79f3621). If the patient is in atrial fibrillation, this pulsating characteristic is lost, but the mitral valve movement can still be identified that helps localizing the atrium. In most instances, a slight rotation to the left is necessary to identify the atrium and mitral valve. The depth of field of the ultrasonic view can be altered. We usually leave it at 4 cm, but if in doubt, the depth of the ultrasonic view can be increased to 7.5 cm, and this will allow viewing the left

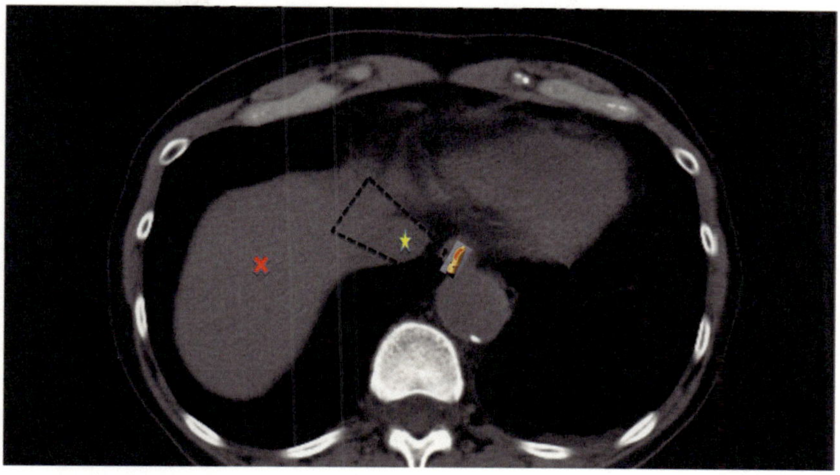

Figure 4.
At the lower end of the esophagus, looking to the right and anteriorly, one can identify the IVC (Yellow star) and liver (red X); the liver also can be seen anteriorly after the scope is passed distally.

ventricle and mitral valve and atrium easily. When using the increased depth on the ultrasonic view, the root of the aorta and the aortic valve are also easily identifiable (**Figure 2**, also see Video at https://mts.intechopen.com/download/index/process/324/authkey/bb9c02ba5640a4d21d4511e0a79f3621). It is necessary to mention here that slight variability exists between patients and moving the scope inferiorly and superiorly or small rotations are necessary to identify all of these structures. The pericardium is an echoic membrane that is almost always separated from the left atrium by a rim of physiologic effusion in this view (a dependent area just posterior to the left atrium in the supine position). When this effusion is big, it can create some confusion to the endoscopist. It is always important to identify the pericardium to avoid puncturing it. Rarely, a mediastinal cyst can occur in this position, which can make the views confusing. Again, increasing the depth on the US screen will help to identify cardiac versus non-cardiac structures. In addition, the use of real time color Doppler will help to separate a cystic structure from a vascular structure, see **Figure 2**. The liver can also be noted and inferior vena cava can be examined too at the distal esophagus just before entering the stomach (**Figure 4**, Video at https://mts.intechopen.com/download/index/process/324/authkey/bb9c02ba5640a4d21d4511e0a79f3621).

6.1 Lymph node stations

In this section, we describe the anatomic definitions according to the eight edition of "Lung Cancer Staging Manual" [25]. We describe "how to reach" the lymph nodal stations, according to our practice. The EUS-B maneuver starts from our point of reference, i.e., the left atrium, in each of the descriptions stated below.

6.1.1 Station seven lymph nodes

Anatomic definition:

Mediastinal node limited by the carina superiorly and upper border of lower lobe bronchus on the left and lower border of the bronchus intermedius on the right.

Conventional name:

Subcarinal lymph nodes.

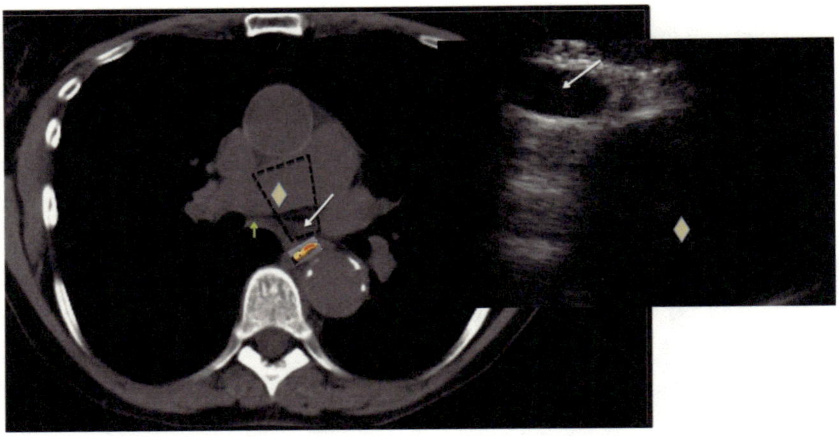

Figure 5.
Rostrally from ***Figure 2****. White arrow shows the pericardial recess, and the diamond is the right pulmonary artery crossing the mediastinum. Note: a slight rotation right will show part of station 7 LN (green arrow).*

EUS location:

This station can be located by slightly pulling the scope rostral above the level of atrium. A slight right or left rotation of the scope is necessary to choose the optimal view of the lymph node and avoid puncturing the great vessels. At the level of station seven, the right pulmonary artery can be identified crossing to the other side of the mediastinum (just deeper to the lymph node on the ultrasound screen, see **Figure 5**).

6.1.2 Stations 8 and 9

Anatomic definition:

Station 8: superiorly limited by the upper border of lower lobe bronchus on the left and lower border of the bronchus intermedius on the right and extends down to the diaphragm.

Station 9: superiorly limited by the inferior pulmonary vein and extends down to the diaphragm. These lymph nodes are located within the pulmonary ligament.

Conventional name:

8: Paraesophageal lymph nodes.

9: Pulmonary ligament lymph nodes.

EUS location:

They are identified by rotating the scope right or left with gently moving it caudally.

Station 9 is identified as any node that associated (in close proximity to) the inferior pulmonary vein and are within the pulmonary ligaments. Station 9 lymph nodes can extend in the pulmonary ligament to the diaphragm, but the only "visible" part of the station is at the junction of the inferior pulmonary vein with the left atrium.

Station 8 lymph nodes are paraesophageal lymph nodes. The upper border is difficult to localize precisely by EUS but in general are the nodes that are on either side of the esophagus below the superior border of the left atrium and extend down to the level of the diaphragm. Of note, both superior pulmonary veins and inferior pulmonary vein on the right are not always identifiable, the left inferior pulmonary vein is almost always identifiable on EUS-B and serves as a landmark for both sides of the mediastinum; it identifies the pulmonary ligament. It is hard to differentiate between level 9 and level 8 near the level of the inferior pulmonary vein. The clinical significance of this differentiation is almost nil, since the presence of metastasis to these lymph nodes from a primary lung cancer indicates N2 if on same side or N3 if the primary cancer is on the other side.

6.1.3 Station 4L

Anatomic definition:

Extends to the upper limits of the aortic arch and down to upper rim of the left main pulmonary artery.

Conventional name:

Left lower paratracheal lymph nodes.

EUS location:

This can be reached with either of two techniques. **First**, from the reference point, the scope can be rotated to the left lateral position then slowly withdrawn until the left pulmonary artery is visualized, if the scope is withdrawn more, the arch of aorta can be visualized. Station 4L is any node that is below the upper border of the arch of aorta in that view and above the upper rim of the main pulmonary artery. The **second** approach involves rotating the scope posteriorly from our reference point anticlockwise; the descending aorta can be seen as a hypoechoic elongated structure. The descending aorta can be followed upward until it starts to disappear. This is the level of the arch, which can be followed through its course at that point by rotating anteriorly (clockwise). Once the arch is identified, advancing the scope caudally will identify the station 4 lymph nodes and left pulmonary artery, see **Figure 6**.

6.1.4 Station 5

Anatomic definition:

Superiorly limited by the lower border of the aortic arch and inferiorly by the upper rim of the left main pulmonary artery. Note that this station is lateral to ligamentum arteriosum, while station 4L is medial to that ligament.

Conventional name:

Subaortic (aorto-pulmonary window) lymph nodes.

EUS location:

This lymph node station can be identified using the same technique for the station 4L. The only difference is that the station 5 lymph nodes are those that are deeper to the ligamentum arteriosum and below the lower rim of the aortic arch. The ligamentum arteriosum, when visible, is identified as an elongated hyperechoic

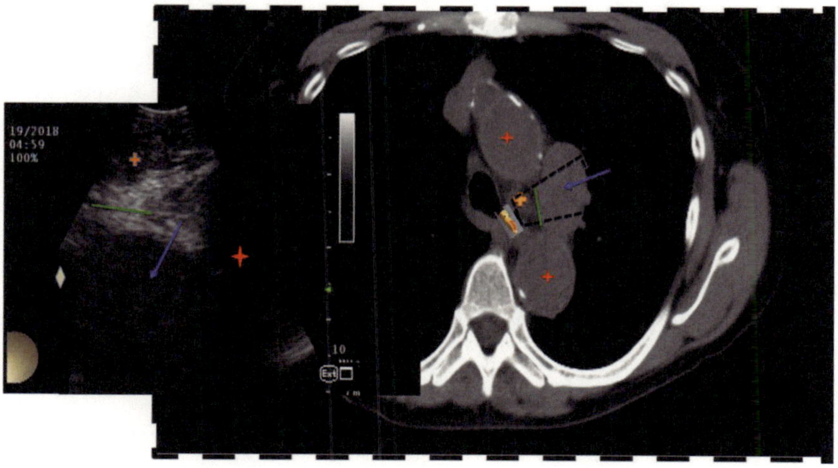

Figure 6.
Red star is the aorta, blue arrow (mass/ LN at station 5), orange cross is station 4L, green is the ligamentum arteriosum separating 4L from station 5. Note: on US view that the ligamentum arteriosum can be seen as dense, hyper-echoic structure connecting the inferior border of aorta to the pulmonary artery.

structure connecting the left pulmonary artery to the aortic arch (**Figure 6**). It is important to mention here that sometimes, one is faced with large lymph nodes or conglomerate of nodes in this position; the differentiation between 5 and 4L can be difficult. In our opinion, both stations carry the same staging implication if positive for lung cancer (both are N2 or N3 disease, never N1) and the clinical benefit of separating the two stations becomes minimal (this issue remains controversial), see **Figure 6**.

Note: Video (https://mts.intechopen.com/download/index/process/324/authkey/bb9c02ba5640a4d21d4511e0a79f3621) shows EUS-B scope looking posteriorly from the reference point identifying the descending aorta; the scope is withdrawn rostral while following the descending aorta. Once it starts to disappear, the arch is reached. At that point, rotation clockwise to follow the arch is performed. Positioned approximately in the middle of the arch, the scope is pushed slightly caudally until the left pulmonary artery is identified. Station 4L and station 5 are between the arch and the pulmonary artery. The former is closer to the probe and the latter is beyond the echogenic ligamentum arteriosum.

6.1.5 Station 2

Anatomic definition:

Superiorly, it is limited by apex of lungs and pleural cavity and upper border of the manubrium on both sides. Station 2R is limited inferiorly by Intersection of caudal margin of the innominate vein and trachea, while on the left (2L) is inferiorly limited by the upper border of the aorta.

Conventional name:

Upper paratracheal.

EUS location:

The 2L station are identified by same maneuvers as station 4L, once the aortic arch is identified, withdrawing the scope to above the aortic arch identifies station 2L location, this station extends all the way up to the level of the manubrium anteriorly and the apex of the lung, both are hard to identify ultrasonographically. Station 2R is slightly different. Station 2R is the lymph node station that is above the level of the brachiocephalic vein and trachea intersection. Once the aortic arch is identified, close attention needs to be paid to the vessels sprouting from it, the most anterior one is the right brachiocephalic artery, this can be followed anteriorly and once sight is lost, it is crossing the trachea. At that point, rotation to the right can be done; station 2R lymph nodes are above that point. It should be noted that this is not an accurate localization (since we cannot identify the BC vein), but it is the best approximation that we could attain.

6.1.6 Station 3p

Anatomic definition:

Limited superiorly by the apex of the lungs and extends inferiorly to the level of the carina.

Conventional name:

Retrotracheal.

EUS location:

From the reference point, one can withdraw the scope until right above the level of station 7. The scope is then turned posteriorly. All posterior lymph nodes (mostly with a slight rotation to the right) are considered 3p up to the upper esophagus.

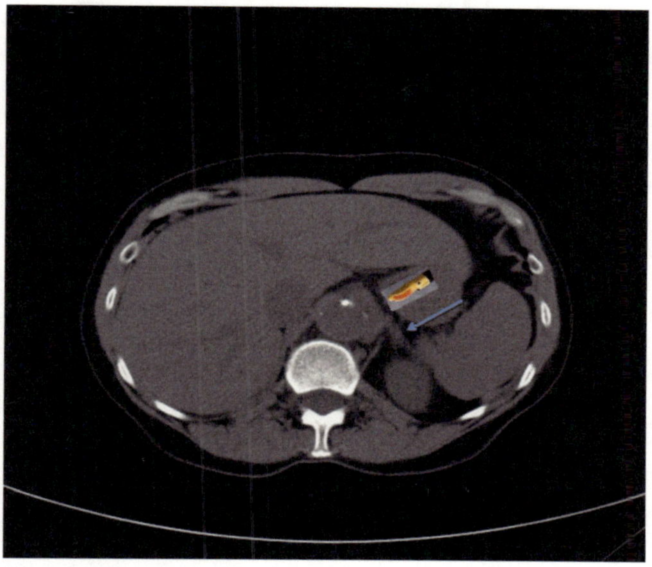

Figure 7.
Once in the stomach, looking posteriorly, one can identify the left adrenal gland (arrow).

6.2 Adrenal glands

Anatomic definition:

The adrenal glands represent the fourth most common site of metastasis for lung cancer. Identifying left adrenal gland is easier than the right. The right adrenal gland cannot be reached by EUS-B. The left adrenal gland is the more common site of adrenal metastasis and easily accessible from the stomach. The endoscopist can identify his presence in the stomach from identification of the stomach folds under US guidance and by visualization of the walls. Several reports of successful biopsy of the left adrenal gland have been described [26, 27], **Figure** 7.

7. Complications

Most of the data available here comes from the literature studying regular endoscopic devices. Endoscopy has proven to be a safe procedure. The rates of complications are probably comparable to that of bronchoscopy. These complications can be classified into two main categories.

7.1 Conscious sedation/anesthesia related

Oxygen desaturation (defined as 4% decrease in hemoglobin saturation below the baseline) can occur in up to 70% of cases without oxygen supplementation [28]. Desaturations occur in both sedated and non-sedated patients. Sedation significantly increases the risk of hypoxia [29]. Supplementary oxygen via nasal cannula reduces the risk [29, 30]. Difficult intubation, therapeutic procedures, increasing age of the patient, and concurrent pulmonary diseases all increase the risk of these events [31, 32]. It is not known if mild desaturations (a drop of 4% on the pulse oximeter) are clinically significant or not. Severe desaturations (pulse oximetry <90%) are less common and can be abolished by the use of supplemental oxygen [28, 32, 33]. The ASGE recommends the use of continuous monitoring devices (pulse oximetry) to monitor for desaturations and correction of hypoxia.

Cardiac complications during endoscopy are also commonly seen and range from mild arrhythmias to severe hypotension and cardiac arrest. Tachycardia is probably the most common arrhythmia seen [28]. A vasovagal response or discomfort from insertion of the scope can be the cause of such a response. Hypotension related to the sedation can also be seen. This can also result from the vasovagal response due to gas insufflation (which is not used during EUS-B).

7.2 Procedure related

Procedure-related complications of esophagoscopy are rare. The major complications of diagnostic esophagoscopy include bleeding, perforation, and infection [28]. Rarely, it would cause strictures or ulcerations. Most of the available literature for EUS-B is from studies evaluating EUS and EUS-FNA of the upper GI tract. Very few studies using EUS-FNA for purpose of lung cancer staging are available. These generally do not comment on rate or types of complications.

Infections can be related to inadequate equipment disinfection, which can be avoided by following the manufacturer guidelines. Another form of infection is the introduction of bacteria to the blood stream or a sterile space (the mediastinum in case of EUS/B-FNA). Episodes of transient bacteremia are a well-known occurrence after upper GI endoscopy (up to 8% of patients) [34]. This is similar for EUS and EUS-FNA according to few reports [35]. Most of these episodes of bacteremia are transient and asymptomatic. Infectious endocarditis is extremely rare ($1–5 \times 10^{-6}$). Prophylactic antibiotics are not necessary for EUS-FNA, unless a cystic mediastinal structure is being sampled [34]. Febrile episodes after endoscopy are also common (about 1%) and are usually transient. Retropharyngeal abscesses have been reported after conventional endoscopy. Isolated reports of benign mediastinal cyst infection have been reported to follow EUS-FNA of these structures [36–38]. The risk for these infections seems to be very small, but one should be aware of the possibility [34]. The ASGE recommends prophylactic antibiotics at time of aspiration and for 3 days.

Perforation of the esophagus with EUS is a known but rare complication (0.03%). Most of the reported data is on radial ultrasonic probes, and limited data exist on the curvilinear probes. It seems that esophageal cancer, stricture, increased age of patient, and an operator with <1 year experience are independent risk factors for perforation [34].

Bleeding occurring can be intra-luminal or extra-luminal. While mild intra-luminal bleeds after EUS-FNA is a relatively common and expected occurrence (up to 4% in one report); extra-luminal bleeding is relatively rare or under-reported due to difficulty in diagnosis [34, 39]. The only reported cases of mediastinal bleeding for sampling of lymph nodes for cancer staging was after a transaortic approach to periaortic lymph nodes (station 6) [40].

8. Contraindications

As for any other technology or procedure, common sense should prevail. If the benefits of the procedure outweigh the risk, then the procedure is probably indicated. We feel that, when present, certain diseases should be avoided and probably considered as contraindications. Esophageal stricture greatly increases the risk of perforation especially that the EUS-B is inserted and maneuvered blindly inside the esophagus. A recent report suggests that the use of EUS-B in the presence of esophageal stricture might be safe. The smaller diameter of the scope enabled the operators to bypass the stricture and attain diagnostic materials in the cases examined [41]. Esophageal varices and portal hypertension should also be considered a contraindication due to the increased risk of bleeding from trauma to the varices. Coagulopathy needs to be corrected and active GI bleeding is a contraindication to this procedure. We believe this procedure should only be performed where back up GI or general surgery expertise is available, in case a complication arises.

9. Summary

In this review, we have tried to lay out an overview of EUS-B. EUS-B is a natural sequel to EBUS for the interventional pulmonologist diagnosing thoracic disease. EUS/B offers access to some nodes not accessible to EBUS, and to paraesophageal masses, which are not also paratracheal. The esophagus is not housed in cartilaginous rings and structures, a factor, which may make some high thoracic lesions accessible to EUS-B alone. As with EBUS, FNA via the esophagus has an extremely low rate of complications. EUS-B does not directly impair respiration. In some cases, EBUS and EUS-B are appropriately performed concurrently, affecting an economy of time, expense, and sedation risks. In short, EUS-B is complementary to EBUS and should be integrated into the diagnostic armamentarium of interventional pulmonology.

Conflict of interest

The authors do not have any conflict of interest to disclose.

Author details

Yousef R. Shweihat* and Shantanu Singh
Section of Pulmonary and Sleep and Critical Care Medicine, Department of Medicine, Marshall University, Huntington, WV, United States of America

*Address all correspondence to: shweihat@marshall.edu

References

[1] Vilmann P, Krasnik M, Larsen SS, Jacobsen GK, Clementsen P. Transesophageal endoscopic ultrasound-guided fine-needle aspiration (EUS-FNA) and endobronchial ultrasound-guided transbronchial needle aspiration (EBUS-TBNA) biopsy: A combined approach in the evaluation of mediastinal lesions. Endoscopy. 2005;**37**(9):833-839

[2] Wallace MB, Pascual JM, Raimondo M, Woodward TA, McComb BL, Crook JE, et al. Minimally invasive endoscopic staging of suspected lung cancer. Journal of the American Medical Association. 2008;**299**(5):540-546

[3] Rintoul RC, Skwarski KM, Murchison JT, Wallace WA, Walker WS, Penman ID. Endobronchial and endoscopic ultrasound-guided real-time fine-needle aspiration for mediastinal staging. The European Respiratory Journal. 2005;**25**(3):416-421

[4] Block MI. Transition from mediastinoscopy to endoscopic ultrasound for lung cancer staging. The Annals of Thoracic Surgery. 2010;**89**(3):885-890

[5] Annema JT, van Meerbeeck JP, Rintoul RC, Dooms C, Deschepper E, Dekkers OM, et al. Mediastinoscopy vs endosonography for mediastinal nodal staging of lung cancer: A randomized trial. Journal of the American Medical Association. 2010;**304**(20):2245-2252

[6] Herth FJ, Krasnik M, Kahn N, Eberhardt R, Ernst A. Combined endoscopic-endobronchial ultrasound-guided fine-needle aspiration of mediastinal lymph nodes through a single bronchoscope in 150 patients with suspected lung cancer. Chest. 2010;**138**(4):790-794

[7] Hwangbo B, Lee GK, Lee HS, Lim KY, Lee SH, Kim HY, et al. Transbronchial and transesophageal fine-needle aspiration using an ultrasound bronchoscope in mediastinal staging of potentially operable lung cancer. Chest. 2010;**138**(4):795-802

[8] Vilmann P, Clementsen PF, Colella S, Siemsen M, De Leyn P, Dumonceau JM, et al. Combined endobronchial and esophageal endosonography for the diagnosis and staging of lung cancer: European Society of Gastrointestinal Endoscopy (ESGE) Guideline, in cooperation with the European Respiratory Society (ERS) and the European Society of Thoracic Surgeons (ESTS). Endoscopy. 2015;**47**(6):545-559

[9] Ko HM, da Cunha Santos G, Darling G, Pierre A, Yasufuku K, Boerner SL, et al. Diagnosis and subclassification of lymphomas and non-neoplastic lesions involving mediastinal lymph nodes using endobronchial ultrasound-guided transbronchial needle aspiration. Diagnostic Cytopathology. Dec 2013;**41**(12):1023-1030. DOI: 10.1002/dc.21741. Epub 2011 May 31

[10] Steinfort DP, Conron M, Tsui A, Pasricha SR, Renwick WE, Antippa P, et al. Endobronchial ultrasound-guided transbronchial needle aspiration for the evaluation of suspected lymphoma. Journal of Thoracic Oncology. 2010;**5**(6):804-809

[11] Kennedy MP, Jimenez CA, Bruzzi JF, Mhatre AD, Lei X, Giles FJ, et al. Endobronchial ultrasound-guided transbronchial needle aspiration in the diagnosis of lymphoma. Thorax. 2008;**63**(4):360-365

[12] Nakajima T, Yasufuku K, Kurosu K, Takiguchi Y, Fujiwara T, Chiyo M, et al. The role of EBUS-TBNA for the diagnosis of sarcoidosis—Comparisons with other bronchoscopic diagnostic modalities. Respiratory Medicine. 2009;**103**(12):1796-1800

[13] Eckardt J, Olsen KE, Jorgensen OD, Licht RB. Minimally invasive

diagnosis of sarcoidosis by EBUS when conventional diagnostics fail. Sarcoidosis, Vasculitis, and Diffuse Lung Diseases. 2010;**27**(1):43-48

[14] Navani N, Booth HL, Kocjan G, Falzon M, Capitanio A, Brown JM, et al. Combination of endobronchial ultrasound-guided transbronchial needle aspiration with standard bronchoscopic techniques for the diagnosis of stage I and stage II pulmonary sarcoidosis. Respirology. 2011;**16**(3):467-472

[15] Hassan T, McLaughlin AM, O'Connell F, Gibbons N, Nicholson S, Keane J. EBUS-TBNA performs well in the diagnosis of isolated thoracic tuberculous lymphadenopathy. American Journal of Respiratory and Critical Care Medicine. 2011;**183**(1):136-137

[16] Lin SM, Ni YL, Kuo CH, Lin TY, Wang TY, Chung FT, et al. Endobronchial ultrasound increases the diagnostic yields of polymerase chain reaction and smear for pulmonary tuberculosis. The Journal of Thoracic and Cardiovascular Surgery. 2010;**139**(6):1554-1560

[17] Steinfort DP, Farmer MW, Irving LB, Jennings BR. Pulmonologist-performed per-esophageal needle aspiration of parenchymal lung lesions using an EBUS bronchoscope: Diagnostic utility and safety. Journal of Bronchology and Interventional Pulmonology. 2017;**24**(2):117-124

[18] Tashi E, Kapisyzi P, Xhemalaj D, Andoni A, Peposhi I. Pancoast tumor approach through oesophagus. Respiratory Medicine Case Reports. 2017;**22**:218-219

[19] Navani N, Nankivell M, Woolhouse I, Harrison RN, Munavvar M, Oltmanns U, et al. Endobronchial ultrasound-guided transbronchial needle aspiration for the diagnosis of intrathoracic lymphadenopathy in patients with extrathoracic malignancy: A multicenter study. Journal of Thoracic Oncology;**6**(9):1505-1509

[20] Al Zoby M, Munn N, Shweihat YR. Esophageal diagnosis of a malignant aspergilloma. Endoscopic Ultrasound. 2017;**6**(3):210-211

[21] Annema JT, Veselic M, Rabe KF. Endoscopic ultrasound-guided fine-needle aspiration for the diagnosis of sarcoidosis. The European Respiratory Journal. 2005;**25**(3):405-409

[22] Puri R, Vilmann P, Sud R, Kumar M, Taneja S, Verma K, et al. Endoscopic ultrasound-guided fine-needle aspiration cytology in the evaluation of suspected tuberculosis in patients with isolated mediastinal lymphadenopathy. Endoscopy. 2010;**42**(6):462-467

[23] Bhaskar N, Shweihat YR, Bartter T. The intubated patient with mediastinal disease—A role for esophageal access using the endobronchial ultrasound bronchoscope. Journal of Intensive Care Medicine. 2014;**29**(1):43-46

[24] Steinfort DP, Irving LB. Patient satisfaction during endobronchial ultrasound-guided transbronchial needle aspiration performed under conscious sedation. Respiratory Care. 2010;**55**(6):702-706

[25] Lababede O, Meziane M, Rice T. Seventh edition of the cancer staging manual and stage grouping of lung cancer: Quick reference chart and diagrams. Chest. 2011;**139**(1):183-189

[26] Meena N, Hulett C, Jeffus S, Bartter T. Left adrenal biopsy using the convex curvilinear ultrasound scope. Respiration. 2015;**89**(1):57-61

[27] Meena N, Hulett C, Patolia S, Bartter T. Exploration under the dome: Esophageal ultrasound with the ultrasound bronchoscope is indispensible. Endoscopic Ultrasound. 2016;**5**(4):254-257

[28] Eisen GM, Baron TH, Dominitz JA, Faigel DO, Goldstein JL, Johanson JF, et al. Complications of upper GI endoscopy. Gastrointestinal Endoscopy. 2002;**55**(7):784-793

[29] Wang CY, Ling LC, Cardosa MS, Wong AK, Wong NW. Hypoxia during upper gastrointestinal endoscopy with and without sedation and the effect of pre-oxygenation on oxygen saturation. Anaesthesia. 2000;**55**(7):654-658

[30] Rozario L, Sloper D, Sheridan MJ. Supplemental oxygen during moderate sedation and the occurrence of clinically significant desaturation during endoscopic procedures. Gastroenterology Nursing. 2008;**31**(4):281-285

[31] Alcain G, Guillen P, Escolar A, Moreno M, Martin L. Predictive factors of oxygen desaturation during upper gastrointestinal endoscopy in nonsedated patients. Gastrointestinal Endoscopy. 1998;**48**(2):143-147

[32] Sarwar S, Alam A, Khan AA. Pulse oximetry during gastrointestinal endoscopic procedures. Journal of the College of Physicians and Surgeons–Pakistan. 2006;**16**(2):97-100

[33] Osinaike BB, Akere A, Olajumoke TO, Oyebamiji EO. Cardiorespiratory changes during upper gastrointestinal endoscopy. African Health Sciences. 2007;7(2):115-119

[34] Adler DG, Jacobson BC, Davila RE, Hirota WK, Leighton JA, Qureshi WA, et al. ASGE guideline: Complications of EUS. Gastrointestinal Endoscopy. 2005;**61**(1):8-12

[35] Janssen J, Konig K, Knop-Hammad V, Johanns W, Greiner L. Frequency of bacteremia after linear EUS of the upper GI tract with and without FNA. Gastrointestinal Endoscopy. 2004;**59**(3):339-344

[36] Ryan AG, Zamvar V, Roberts SA. Iatrogenic candidal infection of a mediastinal foregut cyst following endoscopic ultrasound-guided fine-needle aspiration. Endoscopy. 2002;**34**(10):838-839

[37] Wildi SM, Hoda RS, Fickling W, Schmulewitz N, Varadarajulu S, Roberts SS, et al. Diagnosis of benign cysts of the mediastinum: The role and risks of EUS and FNA. Gastrointestinal Endoscopy. 2003;**58**(3):362-368

[38] Diehl DL, Cheruvattath R, Facktor MA, Go BD. Infection after endoscopic ultrasound-guided aspiration of mediastinal cysts. Interactive Cardiovascular and Thoracic Surgery. 2009;**10**(2):338-340

[39] Affi A, Vazquez-Sequeiros E, Norton ID, Clain JE, Wiersema MJ. Acute extraluminal hemorrhage associated with EUS-guided fine needle aspiration: Frequency and clinical significance. Gastrointestinal Endoscopy. 2001;**53**(2):221-225

[40] von Bartheld MB, Rabe KF, Annema JT. Transaortic EUS-guided FNA in the diagnosis of lung tumors and lymph nodes. Gastrointestinal Endoscopy. 2009;**69**(2):345-349

[41] Buxbaum JL, Eloubeidi MA. Transgastric endoscopic ultrasound (EUS) guided fine needle aspiration (FNA) in patients with esophageal narrowing using the ultrasonic bronchovideoscope. Diseases of the Esophagus. Sep 2011;**24**(7):458-461. DOI: 10.1111/j.1442-2050.2011.01179.x. Epub 2011 Mar 8

Chapter 3

Bronchial Thermoplasty: A New Therapeutic Option in Severe Uncontrolled Asthma

Kumar Sachin

Abstract

Bronchial thermoplasty (BT) is a new endoscopic treatment approved by the US Food and Drug Administration (FDA) in the management of severe refractory asthma involving the delivery of controlled, therapeutic radiofrequency (RF) energy to the airway wall. It is based on the premise of controlling bronchospasm through a reduction of airway smooth muscle (ASM). Several clinical trials have demonstrated improvements in asthma-related quality of life and a reduction in the number of exacerbations following treatment with BT. However, several questions remain regarding the use of BT, mechanism of action, selection of appropriate patients, and long-term effects. Further studies are expected to elucidate the underlying mechanisms that result in these improvements. This chapter discusses key aspects of BT with a focus on the potential clinical effects of this promising procedure. It also offers insight into the barriers to implementing a successful BT program and strategies for overcoming them.

Keywords: severe asthma, bronchial thermoplasty, bronchoscopy, airway smooth muscle

1. Introduction

Asthma is a common condition affecting more than 235 million people worldwide [1]. Asthma is a chronic inflammatory disease characterized by variable airflow obstruction and bronchial hyperreactivity associated with airway remodeling. Clinically, this manifests as recurrent episodes of wheezing, cough, dyspnea, and chest tightness. Asthma treatment as of current standard is based on reducing inflammation with inhaled corticosteroids (ICS) and relaxing airway smooth muscle (ASM) with inhaled bronchodilators along with minimizing exposure to allergic triggers [2]. While most patients achieve symptom control with these strategies, there remains a significant cohort with severe asthma estimated at 5–10% who are more difficult to treat. This group of severe asthmatics, however, is responsible for a disproportionate share of the morbidity associated with the disease. The severe asthma group is responsible for most of the asthma-related healthcare burden, represented by the costs of hospitalizations, ER visits, physician office visits, and use of medications [3–5]. This increased burden of severe asthma reflects the inability of the existing treatment options to adequately control asthma in patients with severe disease.

Severe Asthma is defined by the American Thoracic Society and European Respiratory Society as asthma requiring treatment with high-dose ICS and a second controller medication (and/or systemic corticosteroids) to maintain asthma control [6]. Unfortunately, therapeutic options for patients with severe asthma are limited. Biologic therapy targeting IgE, IL-4 and IL-5 have been of particular interest recently. In the past decade, new therapeutic approaches for asthma have included the use of biological agents, such as omalizumab, a recombinant DNA-derived humanized monoclonal antibody to IgE. However, in patients with severe asthma with no indication for or those lacking a response to omalizumab, the new targeted anti-IL-5 monoclonal antibodies including mepolizumab and reslizumab, have been recently approved [7, 8]. However, they only appear effective in certain subgroups of patients with asthma. Hence, new treatment strategies and approaches are urgently needed for these patients. BT is a novel nonpharmacological therapy which targets ASM in an effort to improve asthma control.

2. Airway smooth muscle in asthma

The airway smooth muscle (ASM) plays significant role in multiple normal processes in the healthy airway, including control of bronchomotor tone, immunomodulation, and extracellular matrix deposition. ASM cells in asthma patients proliferate more rapidly than in non-asthmatic patients, resulting in an increase in smooth muscle mass, with airway narrowing and loss of respiratory function [9]. As a result, the proliferation and differentiation of mesenchymal cells to myofibroblasts increases the deposition of extracellular matrix (ECM) and smooth muscle cells [10]. All of the above modifications, in particular, ASM and ECM deposition, increase the airway wall thickness, which correlates with severity and duration of clinical episodes of asthma [11]. Bronchial remodeling, an increase in ASM, has been shown to be related to clinical and functional severity of asthma [9]. It has been shown that those with fatal asthma have an increased volume of smooth muscle compared with nonfatal asthma [12].

These published findings led to the conclusion that smooth muscle cell alteration is the fundamental structural change that distinguishes severe from moderate asthma, and that phenotypic changes in ASM could contribute to reducing control in subjects with severe asthma [13]. As a result, ASM has become a therapeutic target.

3. Bronchial thermoplasty

BT is a nonpharmacological, novel endoscopic therapy that delivers controlled RF thermal energy to the airway wall as part of a series of three bronchoscopic procedures. It was approved by the US Food and Drug Administration for the treatment of severe persistent asthma in patients aged over 18 years in 2010.It involves application of RF thermal energy to the airways in asthma patients with the goal of ablating the ASM. The first study of BT in human airways involved subjects undergoing lobectomy for known or suspected lung cancer [14].

The current understanding is that BT can denature and destroy ASM and allows the reduction of bronchospasm which in turn results in improved control of the symptoms of severe asthma. Previous canine animal models have demonstrated that BT causes almost complete destruction of ASM with moderate connective tissue deposition when lung tissue has been examined histologically [15].

Several clinical trials have demonstrated the long-term safety and effectiveness of BT in terms of reducing exacerbations of asthma and improving patient quality of life [16].

This chapter will summarize the information on mechanism of action, procedure, efficacy, safety and patient selection, to better understand the path forward for this promising technique.

4. Efficacy data in the short and long term: BT trials to real life

The first randomized clinical trial (RCT) evaluating the efficacy of BT was conducted in 2006 by Cox et al. on 16 patients with stable mild-to-moderate asthma [17]. In general, BT was well tolerated, with most of the procedure-related adverse events occurring in the week following the procedure. Most of the events were mild and transient and resolved spontaneously or required minor changes in medications. There was a significant reduction in airway hyperresponsiveness as reflected by increased PC20 (provocative concentration causing a 20% decline in FEV1). In addition, there was a significant improvement in symptom-free days (47 vs. 73%, $P = 0.015$) and peak expiratory flow rates measured at 12 weeks following BT. Interestingly, there was no change in FEV1 during the 2 years of follow-up. Chest CT was performed at 1 year and 2 years following BT did not reveal any bronchiectasis or parenchymal lung disease [17].

Asthma Intervention Research (AIR) trial was the next major RCT in 2007. AIR included 112 patients with moderate-to-severe asthma (FEV1 between 60 and 85% of predicted) treated with BT [18]. Although, there were no differences in prebronchodilator FEV1 percentage of predicted (72–74.3% vs. 75.8–75.7%, $P = 0.28$) between patients who underwent BT and the control group when compared to their pre-randomization baseline. There was, however, a significant improvement in asthma symptoms as reflected by symptom-free days (40.6 ± 39.7% vs. 17.0 ± 37.9%, $P = 0.005$), scores of the asthma control questionnaire (ACQ) (reduction, 1.2 ± 1.0 vs. 0.5 ± 1.0, $P = 0.001$) and asthma quality of life questionnaire (AQLQ) (1.3 ± 1.0 vs. 0.6 ± 1.1, $P = 0.003$). Moreover, there was a significant reduction in mild exacerbations of asthma and an increase in the morning PEF, in patients treated with BT [18].

In 2007, the Research in Severe Asthma (RISA) designed to evaluate the safety and efficacy of BT in patients with severe, symptomatic asthma was published [19]. This smaller trial included 32 patients (15 randomized to BT) with severe persistent asthma as defined by uncontrolled symptoms despite high-dose ICS and LABA use. Patients in BT arm showed a significant improvement in pre-bronchodilator FEV1. The improvements in ACQ and AQLQ score persisted despite the reduction of OCSs and bronchodilators.

These results were promising, however questions remained over the true efficacy of BT versus potential placebo effect as the RISA and the AIR trials were unblinded [19]. The AIR-2 trial was designed to answer these questions.

5. AIR-2 trial

The largest RCT, AIR2, was a double-blinded, randomized, sham-controlled study included patients who had uncontrolled asthma despite high-dose ICS and a LABA [20]. A total of 190 patients were treated with BT and 98 control patients received sham thermoplasty. The procedure was performed by an unblinded bronchoscopy team and all the assessments and follow-up visits were conducted by

Study	Study population	Study design	Results
Cox et al. [17]	16 patients with mild-to-moderate stable asthma	Non-randomized, prospective study	Significant reduction in airway hyperresponsiveness and increase of symptoms-free days. No changes in FEV1
Cox et al. [18]	112 patients with moderate-to-severe asthma	Randomized, controlled trial	Improvements of asthma symptoms, symptom-free days, and AQLQ and ACQ scores, and reduction in mild exacerbations. No changes in FEV1 and bronchial hyperreactivity
Pavord et al. [19]	32 patients with severe uncontrolled asthma	Randomized, double-blind, parallel-group trial	Significant improvement in FEV1 and ACQ scores. Limitation: effective placebo
Castro et al. [20]	288 patients with severe, uncontrolled asthma	Randomized, double-blind, controlled, multicenter-based trial	Increase of AQLQ score, and reduction of rate of exacerbations, emergency hospital visits, and lost working days
Thomson et al. [21]	69 patients enrolled in the AIR trial	Long-term follow-up study	Significant reduction in airway hyperreactivity and stability of FEV1. No radiological changes
Pavord et al. [22]	14 patients enrolled in RISA trial	Long-term follow-up study	Significant decrease of emergency hospital admissions. No changes of FEV1 value
Wechsler et al. [23]	160 patients enrolled in AIR-2 trial	Long-term follow-up study	Significant decrease of emergency hospital admissions

Abbreviations: FEV1, forced expiratory volume in 1 sec; AQLQ, Asthma Quality of Life Questionnaire; ACQ, Asthma Control Questionnaire; AIR, Asthma Intervention Research; RISA, Research in Severe Asthma.

Table 1.
Summary of clinical trials and long term follow up with BT in asthma.

a blinded team [20]. The primary outcome measure was to evaluate change from baseline in average group mean Asthma Quality of Life Questionnaire (AQLQ) score. In the BT group, a significantly greater proportion had a significant increase in the AQLQ score compared with those who underwent sham bronchoscopy (79 vs. 64%). There was also a meaningful reduction in the number of exacerbations (32% risk reduction), emergency department visits (84% risk reduction) and days lost from school/work (66% risk reduction) in those in the BT arm [20].

The results of these large RCTs are summarized in **Table 1**.

6. Long-term follow up and safety of BT

The earlier large clinical trials of BT showed marked improvements in asthma-related quality of life and a reduction in the number of exacerbations and led to the approval of the use of BT by the FDA in 2010 (**Table 1**). However, long-term safety of BT was largely unaddressed, especially because of early concerns about thermal tissue damage, possible subsequent risk of bronchial stenosis, and bronchomalacia remained to be investigated. Recently, the results from the long-term follow-up of patients enrolled in the AIR, RISA, and AIR-2 trials have provided some clarity in this regard.

From the original study population of patients in the AIR trial, 45 patients treated with BT and 24 control patients were followed for an additional 4 years

(5 years in total) and an additional 2 years (3 years in total) respectively [21]. In comparison to the control subjects, patients who underwent BT had similar rates of adverse respiratory events, oral corticosteroid bursts requirements, hospitalizations, and emergency department visits. Further, patients treated with BT continued to show improvements in airway hyperresponsiveness lasting up to 3 years, suggesting the long-term efficacy of the procedure [21].

A long-term follow up of the patients with BT included in the RISA study, performed for a total of 5 years, showed a significant decline in emergency visits and hospitalizations for an exacerbation of asthma, and no further deterioration of FEV1 [22].

Similarly, in the AIR-2 follow up study, patients were also monitored for another 4 years to evaluate the long-term effects of BT [23]. Patients treated with BT showed a definite decrease in severe exacerbations of asthma and emergency hospital visits [23]. Interestingly, a recent large retrospective study of patients with persistent asthma suggests constant exacerbation frequency despite continued high-intensity therapy with high doses of ICS and LABAs [24]. Therefore, long-term comparative head to head safety studies for the use of BT in the treatment of asthma are nevertheless required in future also.

7. Patient selection for bronchial thermoplasty

Currently, BT is approved for patients with uncontrolled severe persistent asthma despite the use of an inhaled corticosteroid and LABA. As per the recent Global Initiative for Asthma (GINA) guidelines, it has been suggested that "for highly-selected adult patients with uncontrolled asthma despite use of recommended therapeutic regimens and referral to an asthma specialty center, BT is a potential treatment option" (Grade B evidence) [25]. In general, BT remains contraindicated in patients with a pacemaker, internal defibrillator, or any implantable electronic device [25].

Prior to consideration of BT, patients should undergo a focused evaluation to ensure that the diagnosis of severe asthma is correct, treatment is optimized, and comorbid conditions are treated. A thorough history and detailed physical examination constitute the next step. In addition, workup as necessary to exclude an alternative diagnosis, such as sarcoidosis, cystic fibrosis (CF), other non-CF bronchiectatic lung disease, alpha-1 antitrypsin deficiency, and chronic obstructive pulmonary disease (COPD) should also be carried out [26]. In general, full pulmonary function testing as well as a high-resolution CT scan of the lungs is also desirable. Before labeling it as severe asthma, the inhaler technique and adherence are also evaluated rigorously, as corrective interventions have shown to improve asthma control [27].

8. BT procedure

BT is based on the principle of endobronchial controlled delivery of RF thermal energy to modify the structure of the airway wall thereby reducing the amount of ASM with a device called the Alair BT System (Boston Scientific, Marlborough, MA, USA). A bronchoscope with a disposable catheter with a diameter of 2.0 mm in the operating channel is used to obtain better visualization and complete treatment of subsegmental bronchi [17]. The distal tip of the catheter has an expandable four-electrode basket, through which 65°C radio frequencies are delivered in order to visible bronchial areas sequentially [17]. The correct order involves the right lower lobe (first session) then left lower lobe (second session), followed by both upper lobes (third session). The right middle lobe is generally not treated because of the remote possibility of obstruction and right middle lobe syndrome. A typical BT session lasts about 30–45 min.

The entire visible length of each bronchus is treated with each pulse targeting a 5 mm section of bronchus between 3 and 10 mm in diameter, starting at the periphery and moving proximally. On an average the full treatment consists of 30–70 activations per lobe, up to 44 for the right lower lobe, 47 for the left lower lobe and 60 for the upper lobes [21]. Successful BT comprises three procedures performed at 20 day intervals [17]. Mild bronchoconstriction, mucous hypersecretion, and minor bleeding related to superficial trauma are the most commonly encountered complications. Patients are given systemic corticosteroids and nebulized. Bronchodilators prior and after the procedure to minimize the complications in the post procedure setting.

BT should be performed by an experienced bronchoscopist in an adequate setting with appropriate clinical monitoring and the facility and expertise to address any potential post-intervention complications. Mayse et al. has described the appropriate assessment and monitoring of the patient before, during and after the procedure [28].

9. What are the current guidelines regarding bronchial thermoplasty?

As per the current European Respiratory Society and American Thoracic Society (ERS/ATS) guidelines BT is recommended in adults with severe refractory asthma, despite optimal therapy, in the context of an institutional review board-approved independent systematic registry, or for use in a clinical study only [29]. A recent Cochrane Database systematic review also has the same recommendation and highlights the need for further studies on BT to determine the mechanisms of action in patients with different phenotypes of asthma [30]. Interestingly the BT Global Registry, a 2 year observational study is expected to provide new and valuable data on BT, is currently recruiting patients [31].

10. Pharmacoeconomics of bronchial thermoplasty

BT is an expensive procedure, but recent studies have shown that the obvious high cost may be at least partially balanced by the reduction in costs due to decrease in acute exacerbations of asthma requiring emergency department visits and the effects of improved quality of life for patients [32]. A subsequent study has confirmed that BT has a 60% chance to be more cost effective as compared with omalizumab and standard therapy on the willingness-to pay of $100,000/quality-adjusted life year [33]. Zein and colleagues also concluded that BT is a cost effective intervention in patients with asthma at high risk of exacerbations [34]. However, a study carried out in Singapore found that BT is not cost effective compared with optimized asthma therapy unless the cost of the procedure is decreased so as to make it more cost effective [35].

11. Conclusions

BT is the only FDA approved nonpharmacological treatment available for severe asthma patients. In contrast to therapies for asthma targeting the underlying inflammatory response, BT specifically targets the ASM. Recent clinical trials have established its safety, ability to improve quality of life and reduction in exacerbations in patients with severe asthma. However, the exact mechanisms that underlie these improvements seen with BT remain at best still poorly understood. Future studies on the mechanism of action of BT, including phenotyping of patients and treatment approaches in identifying the patients most likely to respond to this therapy are expected to solve the existing conundrum.

Conflict of interest

The author does not disclose any conflict of interest.

Author details

Kumar Sachin
Pulmonology and Critical Care Medicine, Sakra World Hospital, Bangalore, India

*Address all correspondence to: sachin.drk@gmail.com

References

[1] World Health Organization. Chronic Respiratory Disease, Asthma. Available from: www.who.int/respiratory/asthma/en/

[2] Mitzner W. Airway smooth muscle: The appendix of the lung. American Journal of Respiratory and Critical Care Medicine. 2004;**169**:787-790

[3] Godard P, Chanez P, Siraudin L, Nicoloyannis N, Duru G. Costs of asthma are correlated with severity: A 1-yr prospective study. The European Respiratory Journal. 2002; **19**(1):61-67

[4] Ivanova JI, Bergman R, Birnbaum HG, Colice GL, Silverman RA, McLaurin K. Effect of asthma exacerbations on health care costs among asthmatic patients with moderate and severe persistent asthma. The Journal of Allergy and Clinical Immunology. 2012;**129**(5):1229-1235

[5] Moore WC, Bleecker ER, Curran-Everett D, et al. Characterization of the severe asthma phenotype by the national heart, lung, and blood institutes severe asthma research program. The Journal of Allergy and Clinical Immunology. 2007;**119**(2):405-413

[6] Chung KF, Wenzel SE, Brozek JL, et al. International ERS/ATS guidelines on definition, evaluation and treatment of severe asthma. The European Respiratory Journal. 2014;**43**(2):343-373

[7] Menzella F, Lusuardi M, Galeone C, Taddei S, Facciolongo N, Zucchi L. Mepolizumab for severe refractory eosinophilic asthma: Evidence to date and clinical potential. Therapeutic Advances in Chronic Disease. 2016;**7**(6): 260-277

[8] Máspero J. Reslizumab in the treatment of inadequately controlled asthma in adults and adolescents with elevated blood eosinophils: Clinical trial evidence and future prospects. Therapeutic Advances in Respiratory Disease. 2017;**11**(8):311-325

[9] Pascual RM, Peters SP. Airway remodeling contributes to the progressive loss of lung function in asthma: An overview. The Journal of Allergy and Clinical Immunology. 2005; **116**:477-486

[10] Noble PB, Pascoe CD, Lan B, et al. Airway smooth muscle in asthma: Linking contraction and mechanotransduction to disease pathogenesis and remodeling. Pulmonary Pharmacology & Therapeutics. 2014;**29**(2):96-107

[11] Nair P, Martin JG, Cockcroft DC, et al. Airway hyperresponsiveness in asthma: Measurement and clinical relevance. The Journal of Allergy and Clinical Immunology. In Practice. 2017; **5**(3):649.e2-659.e2

[12] Carroll N, Elliot J, Morton A, et al. The structure of large and small airways in nonfatal and fatal asthma. The American Review of Respiratory Disease. 1993;**147**:405-410

[13] Panettieri RA Jr, Kotlikoff MI, Gerthoffer WT, et al. National Heart, Lung, and Blood Institute. Airway smooth muscle in bronchial tone, inflammation, and remodeling: Basic knowledge to clinical relevance. American Journal of Respiratory and Critical Care Medicine. 2008;**177**(3): 248-252

[14] Miller JD, Cox G, Vincic L, Lombard CM, Loomas BE, Danek CJ. A prospective feasibility study of bronchial thermoplasty in the human airway. Chest. 2005;**127**(6):1999-2006

[15] Danek CJ, Lombard CM, Dungworth DL, et al. Reduction in airway hyperresponsiveness to methacholine by the application of RF

energy in dogs. Journal of Applied Physiology (Bethesda, MD: 1985). 2004; **97**(5):1946-1953

[16] Trivedi A, Pavord ID, Castro M. Bronchial thermoplasty and biological therapy as targeted treatments for severe uncontrolled asthma. The Lancet Respiratory Medicine. 2016;**4**(7): 585-592

[17] Cox G, Miller JD, McWilliams A, Fitzgerald JM, Lam S. Bronchial thermoplasty for asthma. American Journal of Respiratory and Critical Care Medicine. 2006;**173**(9):965-969

[18] Cox G, Thomson NC, Rubin AS, et al. AIR trial study group. Asthma control during the year after bronchial thermoplasty. The New England Journal of Medicine. 2007;**356**(13):1327-1337

[19] Pavord ID, Cox G, Thomson NC, et al. RISA trial study group. Safety and efficacy of bronchial thermoplasty in symptomatic, severe asthma. American Journal of Respiratory and Critical Care Medicine. 2007;**176**(12):1185-1191

[20] Castro M, Rubin AS, Laviolette M, et al. AIR2 trial study group. Effectiveness and safety of bronchial thermoplasty in the treatment of severe asthma: A multicenter, randomized, double-blind, sham-controlled clinical trial. American Journal of Respiratory and Critical Care Medicine. 2010;**181**(2): 116-124

[21] Thomson NC, Rubin AS, Niven RM, et al. AIR trial study group. Long-term (5 year) safety of bronchial thermoplasty: Asthma intervention research (AIR) trial. BMC Pulmonary Medicine. 2011;**11**:8

[22] Pavord ID, Thomson NC, Niven RM, et al. Research in severe asthma trial study group. Safety of bronchial thermoplasty in patients with severe refractory asthma. Annals of Allergy, Asthma & Immunology. 2013;**111**(5): 402-407

[23] Wechsler ME, Laviolette M, Rubin AS, et al. Asthma intervention research 2 trial study group. Bronchial thermoplasty: Long-term safety and effectiveness in patients with severe persistent asthma. The Journal of Allergy and Clinical Immunology. 2013; **132**(6):1295-1302

[24] Schatz M, Meckley LM, Kim M, Stockwell BT, Castro M. Asthma exacerbation rates in adults are unchanged over a 5-year period despite high-intensity therapy. The Journal of Allergy and Clinical Immunology. In Practice. 2014;**2**(5):570-574. e1

[25] Global Initiative for Asthma (GINA) [Internet]. Global Strategy for Asthma Management and Prevention. Available from: https://ginasthma.org/2018-gina-report-global-strategy-for-asthma-management-and-prevention/ [Accessed December 25, 2018]

[26] Robinson DS, Campbell DA, Durham SR, et al. Asthma and Allergy Research Group of the National Heart and Lung Institute. Systematic assessment of difficult-to-treat asthma. The European Respiratory Journal. 2003;**22**(3):478-483

[27] Gamble J, Stevenson M, Heaney LG. A study of a multi-level intervention to improve non-adherence in difficult to control asthma. Respiratory Medicine. 2011;**105**(9):1308-1315

[28] Mayse ML, Laviolette M, Rubin AS. Clinical pearls for bronchial thermoplasty. Journal of Bronchology. 2007;**14**:115-123

[29] Wenzel SE. Asthma phenotypes: The evolution from clinical to molecular approaches. Nature Medicine. 2012; **18**(5):716-725

[30] Torrego A, Solà I, Munoz AM, et al. Bronchial thermoplasty for moderate or severe persistent asthma in adults. Cochrane Database of Systematic Reviews. 2014;**3**:CD009910

[31] Boston Scientific. Bronchial Thermoplasty Global Registry (BT Registry). 2014. Availablefrom: https://clinicaltrials.gov/ct2/show/NCT02104856 [Accessed December 25, 2018]. ClinicalTrials.gov identifier: NCT02104856

[32] Menzella F, Zucchi L, Piro R, Galeone C, Castagnetti C, Facciolongo N. A budget impact analysis of bronchial thermoplasty for severe asthma in clinical practice. Advances in Therapy. 2014;**31**(7):751-761

[33] Zafari Z, Sadatsafavi M, Marra CA, Chen W, FitzGerald JM. Cost-effectiveness of bronchial thermoplasty, omalizumab, and standard therapy for moderate-to-severe allergic asthma. PLoS One. 2016;**11**(1):e0146003

[34] Zein JG, Menegay MC, Singer ME, et al. Cost effectiveness of bronchial thermoplasty in patients with severe uncontrolled asthma. The Journal of Asthma. 2016;**53**:194-200

[35] Nguyen HV, Bose S, Mital S, et al. Is bronchial thermoplasty cost-effective as treatment for problematic asthma patients? Singapore's perspective on a global model. Respirology. 2017;**22**(6):1102-1109

Chapter 4

Virtual Bronchoscopy for Tumors and Traumatic Lesions of the Airways

Kotlyarov Peter Mikhaylovich

Abstract

The given MSCT of 26 patients with tumoral damage of a trachea is analyzed. Data of MSCT of 61 patients with tumoral damage of bronchial tubes of primary and secondary genesis and hyperplastic lymph nodes are analyzed. In the analysis, a comprehensive analysis of the native, post-processing data and volumetric reconstructions allows more fully appreciating the nature of the changes, the topography, the extent and prevalence of neoplastic lesions tracheobronchial system. Differential diagnostics of benign and malignant lesions are conducted especially in the stenotic lesions when execution of bronchofibroscopy was impossible. Virtual bronchoscopy (VB) MSCT allowed determining the presence of a complete or partial rupture of the main bronchus, its distance to the bifurcation of the trachea, the state of the collapsed lung, the presence of fluid in the hemithorax, and secondary changes in the bone structures of the chest. The VB played an important role in monitoring the adequacy of reconstructive measures on the damaged bronchus, excluding the occurrence of postoperative stenosis. Virtual bronchoscopy of multispiral computed tomography with the capabilities of multiplanar and volumetric reconstructions and post-processing image processing is an optimal noninvasive method for determining the traumatic lesion of the main bronchi and monitoring the success of the reconstructive surgical manual

Keywords: virtual bronchoscopy, multislice computed tomography, tumor airways, traumatic bronchus rupture

1. Virtual bronchoscopy multislice computer tomography in diagnostics of neoplastic lesions of the tracheobronchial systems

1.1 Introduction

The defeat of the tracheobronchial system (TBS) by cancer is 17.8% in men and 3.7% in women [1]. Trachea, in addition to primary tumors, can be affected a second time with cancers of the esophagus, thyroid, and lungs. A number of benign tumors grow inside the lumen of the trachea and bronchi, causing a violation of the lung ventilation. Large bronchi may be secondarily affected in the central and peripheral forms of lung cancer [2–4]. The introduction of clinical practice of multispiral computed tomography (MSCT) clinical practice, new technologies of data collection, and post-processing image processing allowed developing a program of

IntechOpen

3D reconstruction of the tracheobronchial system (TBS) with the ability to view its inner surface in real-time virtual bronchoscopy (VB) [2–16]. In addition to VB methods such as minimum and maximum intensity (MinIP, MIP) images, the mode of shaded surfaces—VTR allow to assess the state of the outer wall of the TBS, the relationship with adjacent organs and tissues [4, 5, 8, 16]. Comparison of the data of FBS and VB of the zone of interest showed their coincidence in the evaluation of the macrostructure of the bronchial lumen, the presence of intrabronchial tumor masses, and their type and localization [4, 9, 12]. In addition, the study of the bronchus distal to the stenosis at bronchoscopy is difficult and VB is the only method giving the possibility to evaluate the macrostructure of the bronchus beyond the area of narrowing [2, 5, 16]. The restrained attitude to VB of radiologists of foreign countries at the initial stage of data accumulation was replaced by a wide application of the method in clinical practice, as indicated by a significant increase in publications in recent years [2, 3, 7–13]. The purpose of the study is to clarify the concept of VB techniques and their role in improving the diagnostic information content of CT in the diagnosis and prevalence of neoplastic lesions of TBS.

1.2 Materials and methods of research

The MSCT data of 26 patients with tracheal tumor lesions were analyzed. Adenoid cystic cancer of the trachea was observed in 10 (32, 25%) patients, squamous cell in 6 (of 19.35%) patients, and neoplastic lesions of the trachea in 5 patients; the process has spread outside the body wall infiltrating the surrounding tissue. Of 10 (32, 25%) patients who had benign tumor, 4 had adenoma of the trachea, 3 had polyp, and 3 had papillomatosis. We analyzed patients' data of 61 MSCT with a neoplastic lesion of the bronchi of primary and secondary origin and hyperplastic lymph nodes. Lung cancer took place in 35 (57.37%) patients, metastatic lung damage and lymph nodes were observed in 5 (8.19%), and post-inflammatory hyperplasia of the lymph node adjacent to the bronchus in 4 (6.55%). In 17 (27, 86%) patients, benign bronchial formations of adenoma—8, polyposis—5 and papillomatosis—4 were revealed.

The diagnosis was verified in all patients in the process of material sampling in FBS and morphology according to the results of surgery.

MSCT was performed on 128-slice computed tomography company "GE Healthcare", model "Optima CT 660". Post-processing data processing, obtaining virtual bronchograms, and 3D imaging were performed at the workstation"Optima CT 660". Постпроцессинговая обработка данных, получение виртуальных бронхограмм. 3D изображений проводилась на рабочей станции Advantage Workstation (GE). Toshiba Aquilion 16 (16-slice) and Aquilion ONE (320-slice) according to the previously described method [4–6, 26]. A comparative analysis of the value of different methods of MSCT VB in determining the lesion of TBS showed the need to use them in a complex for the full characteristics of both the intraluminal part of the trachea, carina, the main bronchi, and the outer wall in the images of the minimum (MinIP) and maximum intensity (MIP). For the reconstruction of 3D data in the images of virtual bronchoscopy, the technique of three-dimensional modeling was used, which produced a three-dimensional array with the display of the inner and the outer surface of the bronchi. Based on these data, a VB examination of the tracheobronchial tree was performed using VB fly-through method and volumetric reconstruction of the lung and its structures. In order to obtain the outer surface of the lung, trachea, or bronchi, the technique of obtaining an image of shaded surfaces and volume conversion was used. The complex analysis necessarily includes the data of native MSCT, the results of which allow avoiding false positive and negative conclusions in the presence of mucus and scar changes in the TBS.

1.3 Results of a research

Data of CT VB of 16 patients with cancer of the trachea were analyzed. At VB tumor mass spreading inside the body lumen was multinodular masses presented heterogeneous density and narrowing the lumen of the organ. The tumor was localized on the wall of the trachea with a wide base, spreading along it or circularly. The tracheal rings of the affected area were not visualized. Followed by multiplanar image reconstruction in MinIP mode, shaded surfaces and volume data transformations allowed visualizing the distribution of neoplastic lesions in the wall of the trachea, the length and volume of the lesion, and the degree of overlap of the organ lumen (**Figure 1**). In 11 patients, the tumor was localized within the tissues of the organ, without infiltrating the surrounding tissue, and in 5 patients, the tracheal wall sprouted and spread to the mediastinal tissue and esophagus (1 patient). In 6 out of 11 patients, the outer edge of the wall had a flat surface and the tumor process spread mainly along the inner surface of the organ, without infiltrating the wall. Thickening of the tracheal wall was observed in five patients, indicating its tumor infiltration. The nonorgan part of the tumor was heterogeneous and multi-nodular, without clear contours with the surrounding tissue. Tumors of the trachea chaotically accumulated a contrast material during bolus contrast enhancement. Followed by multiplanar reconstruction in MIP and MinIP modes, an unorganized component of the trachea cancer was clearly identified. Signs of esophageal germination were compression, overlapping of its lumen, and dilation above the site of infiltration (one patient). Increased regional lymph nodes (diameter 13–17 mm) were additionally determined in five patients, indicating a high degree of probability of metastatic lesions. This MSCT VB did not allow determining the morphological variant of malignant lesions and the state of the tracheal mucosa of the affected area and intact areas.

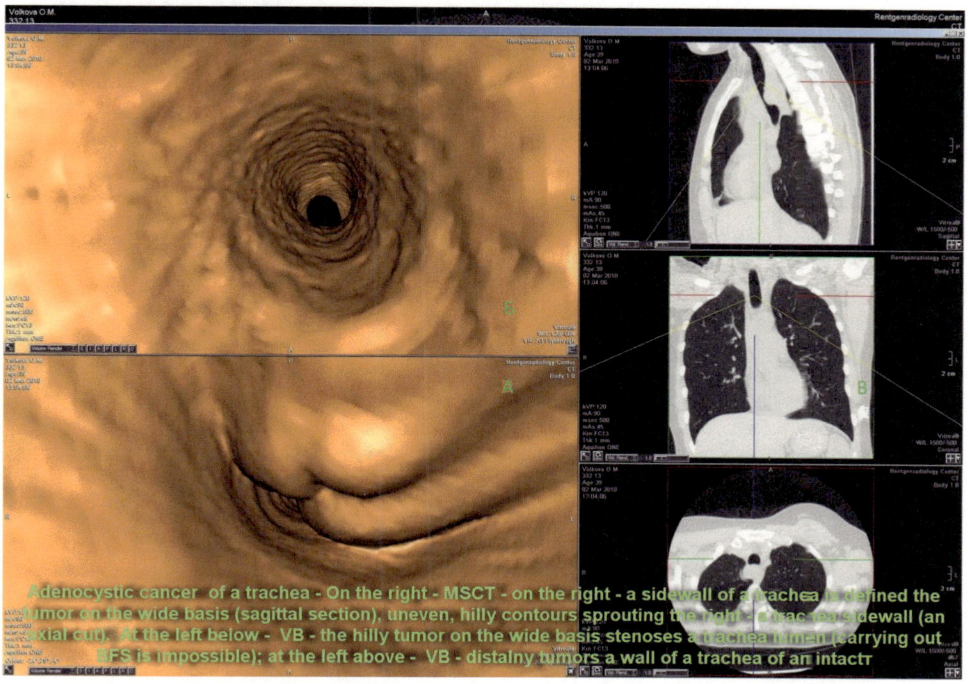

Figure 1.
AQ-Adenocystic cancer of a trachea – On the right – MSCT – on the right – a sidewall of a trachea is defined the tumor on the wide basis (sagittal section), uneven, hilly contours sprouting the right – a trachea sidewall (an axial cut). At the left below – VB – the hilly tumor on the wide basis stenoses a trachea lumen (carrying out BFS is impossible); at the left above – VB – distalny tumors a wall of a trachea of an intact.

The MSCT data of 10 patients with benign tracheal formations were analyzed. Benign formations were characterized by a smooth surface, homogeneous internal structure, no infiltration of the wall, and the destruction of the cartilage of the trachea. Benign tumor of the trachea performed into the lumen of it making its lumen narrowed (**Figure 2a, b**). Focal changes emanating from the exterior pushed them to the opposite side without narrowing of lumen and signs of infiltration of the exterior wall.

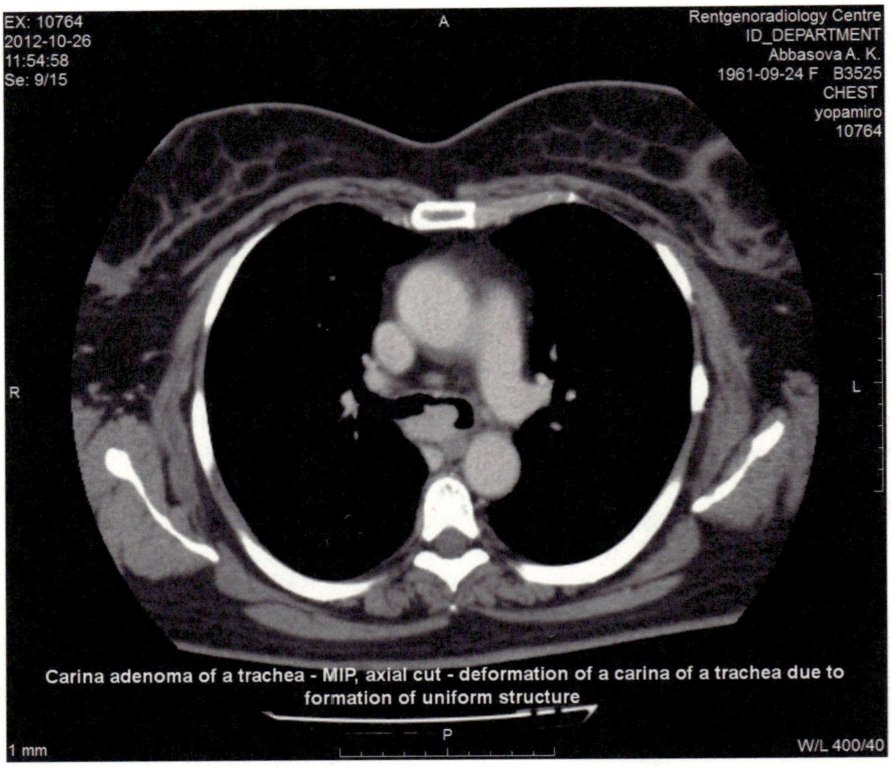

a

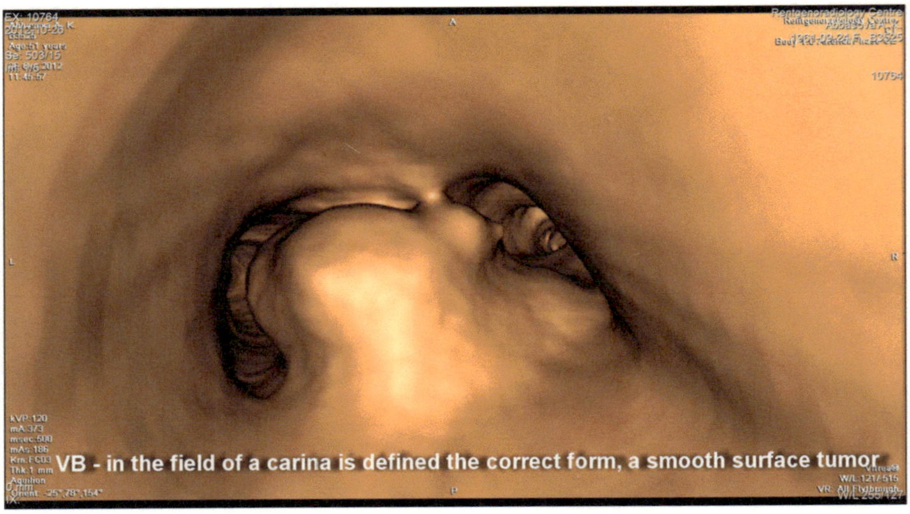

b

Figure 2.
a. Carina adenoma of a trachea – MIP, axial cut – deformation of a carina of a trachea due to formation of uniform structure. b. VB – in the field of a carina is defined the correct form, a smooth surface tumor.

With growth in the direction of the esophagus, the latter was also pushed aside by the formation without signs of its infiltration. Papillomatosis, polyps manifested by visualization of smooth, on the peduncle, the correct form coming from the mucous linear structures localized on the side wall of the trachea (**Figure 3**).

As shown by the combined analysis of native MSCT data and VB techniques (fly-through, MinIP, MIP, and 3D reconstruction), this approach is highly effective in the predictive test of the nature of both primary and secondary organ damage. Benign formations (adenoma, polyp, and others) were characterized by the presence of peduncles, linking the formation and mucous trachea, the wall of which was not thickened or infiltrated. The benign one went out into the lumen of the trachea. It had the right shape, smooth surface, and homogeneous structure. Secondary displacements of the trachea by benign processes emanating from the mediastinum and the esophagus are manifested by the displacement of the organ to the opposite side from the formation, without signs of infiltration of the wall.

Thus, the signs of malignancy tumors of the trachea were wide base and destraction of the adjacent cartilage structures, a rough bumpy surface, infiltration of the wall of the trachea in length, the output of the process beyond the body with tissue infiltration in the mediastinum, spreading to the esophagus. Additional signs of malignancy of changes were visualizations of enlargement of regional lymph nodes.

The data of MSCT VB in 35 patients with lung cancer were analyzed. Three variant neoplastic lesions of the bronchi, mostly peribronchial, intrabronchial, and a combined form of infiltration were observed. As a result of the study, according to the methods of VB fly-through, the leading method of determining the macrostructure and the border of the intrabronchial lesion that were inside the lumen of the bronchus, multinodal, polypoid masses were visualized, usually located on a wide base, narrowing the bronchus down to complete obstruction (**Figure 4a, b**).

The cartilaginous structures of the bronchus in the affected area were not visualized. The distribution of the lesions in the area of the branching of the bronchi last

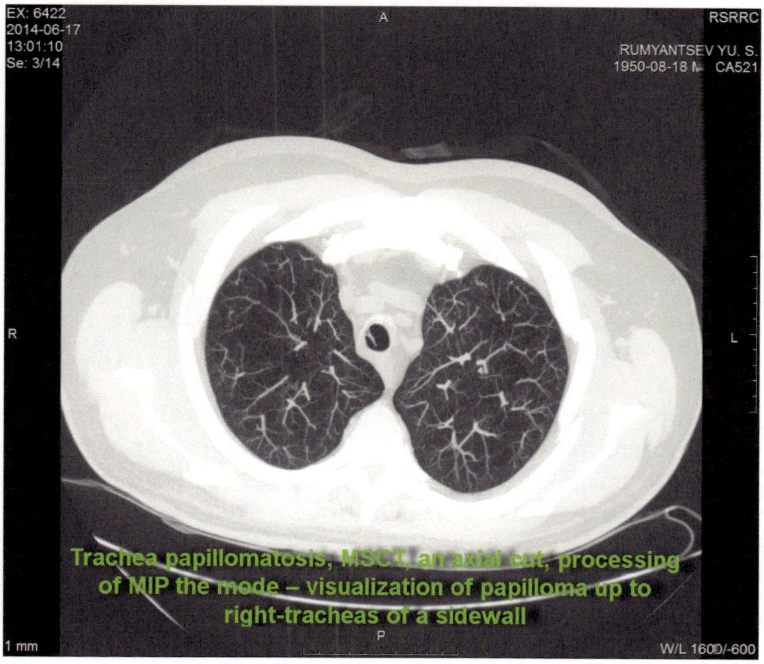

Figure 3.
Trachea papillomatosis, MSCT, an axial cut, processing of MIP the mode – visualization of papilloma up to right-tracheas of a sidewall.

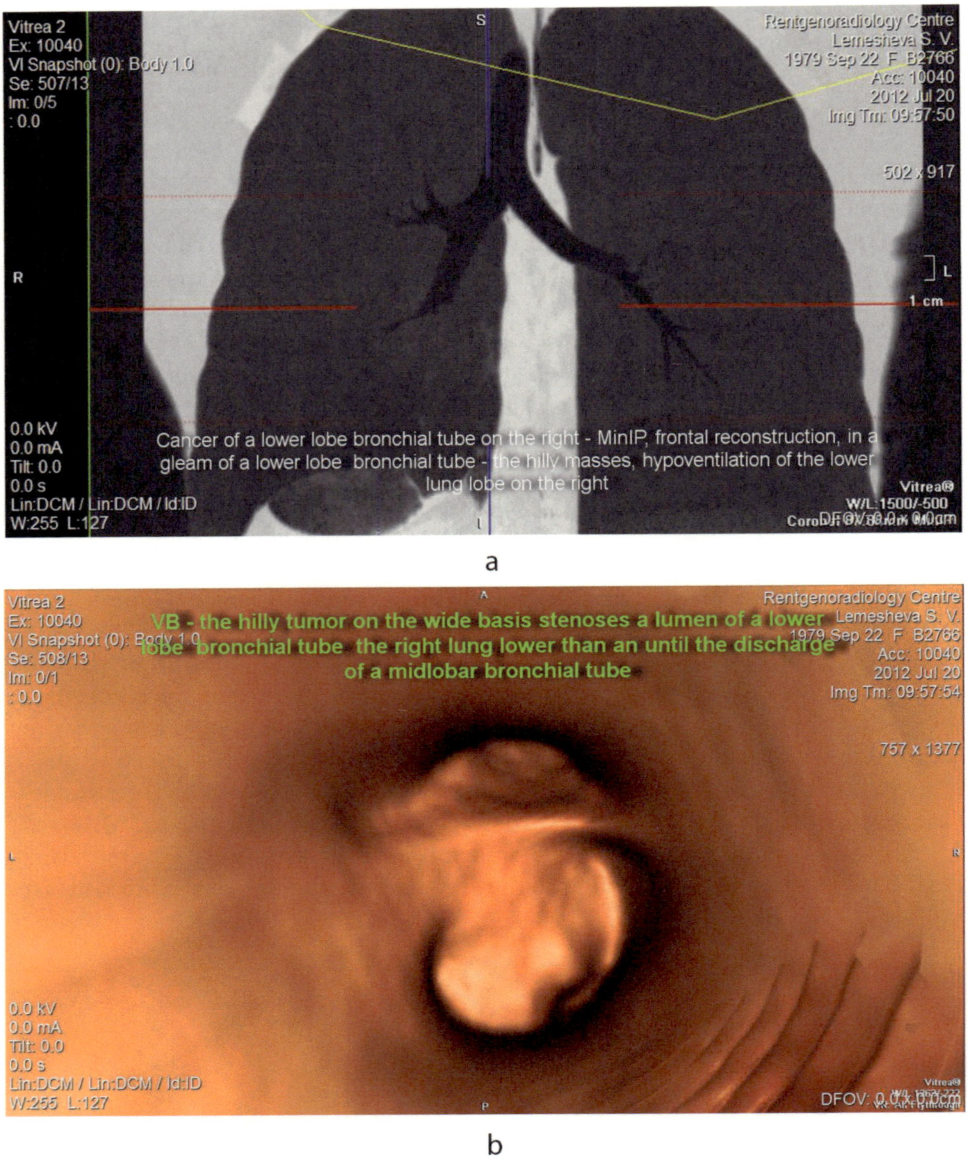

Figure 4.
a. Cancer of a lower lobe bronchial tube on the right – MinIP, frontal reconstruction, in a gleam of a lower lobe bronchial tube – the hilly masses, hypoventilation of the lower lung lobe on the right. b. VB – the hilly tumor on the wide basis stenoses a lumen of a lower lobe bronchial tube the right lung lower than an until the discharge of a midlobar bronchial tube.

lost "pointed" appearance and grew deformed. Carina of the trachea with peribronchial spread the tumor from smooth and it turned into tumor growths covered with shapeless structure. Image of the trachea and bronchi in MIP and MinIP modes and 3D volumetric reconstructions completed the picture WB flythrough, allowing to evaluate the association of intrabronchial mass with pulmonary part of the tumor, and thus, to obtain a holistic view of the prevalence of lung cancer (**Figure 5a, b**).

In peribronchial infiltration (four patients with central cancer), semiotic signs in the mode of MinIP were visualized with varying degrees of local narrowing of the bronchial lumen. The transition of a changed plot of pathologically unchanged tissue of the bronchus was a border infiltration and was a "bayonet-like" extension of the lumen. The analysis showed the presence of sub-variants of peribronchial

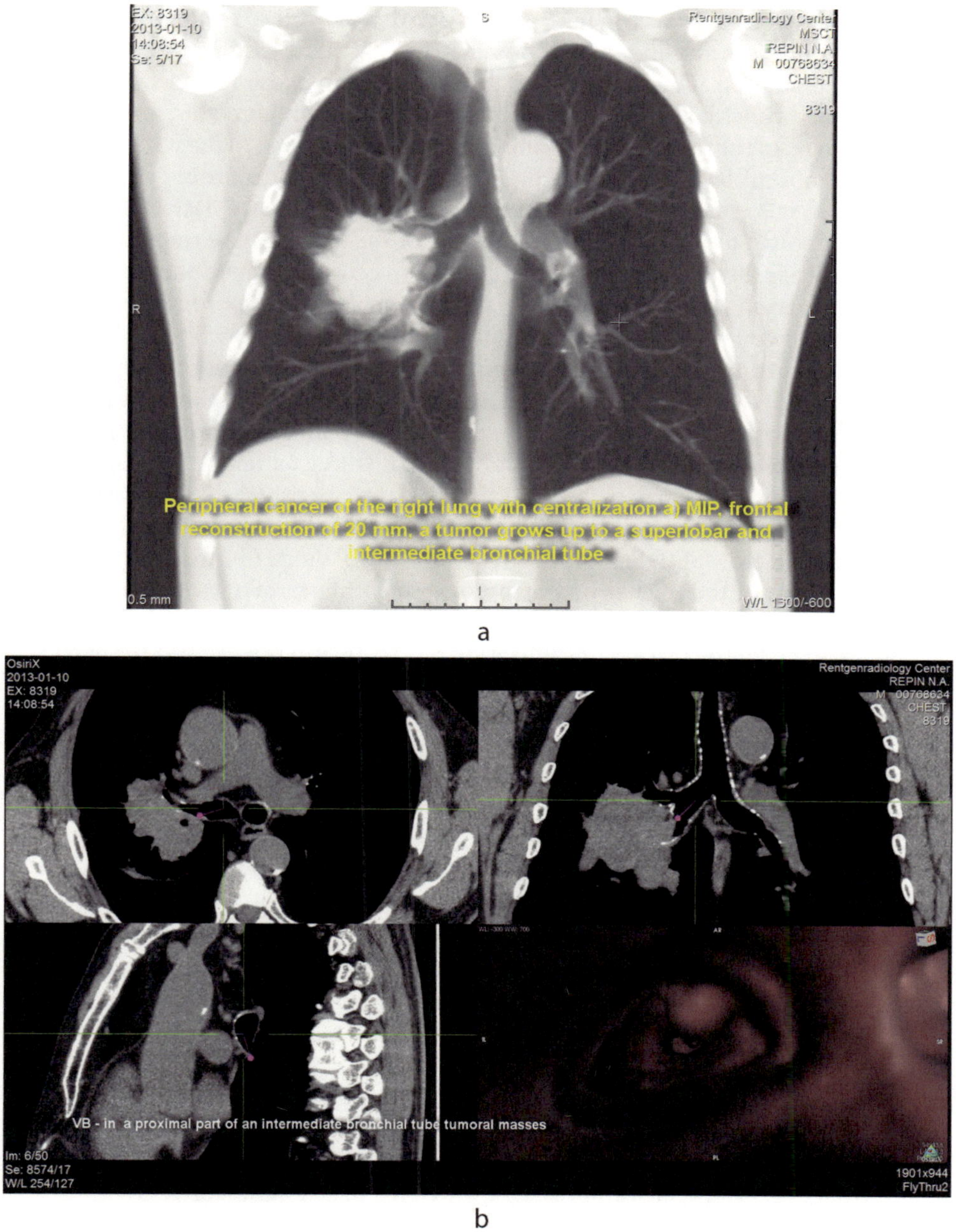

Figure 5.
a. Peripheral cancer of the right lung with centralization a) MIP, frontal reconstruction of 20 mm, a tumor grows up to a superlobar and intermediate bronchial tube. b. VB – in a proximal part of an intermediate bronchial tube tumoral masses.

tumor growth—circular, when they infiltrated all the walls of the bronchi and focal-segmental, in which the tumor struck one of the walls of the bronchus. Method VB fly-through was detected in this group of patients, along with narrowing of the lumen of the bronchus and the disappearance of the rosary-like structure of the bronchi due to infiltration of the cartilaginous structures.

The mixed variant of TBS infiltration was characterized by a combination of symptoms of one and two variants of VB (six patients with central and two peripheral cancer). In addition to intrabronchial component of the tumor, peribronchial growth was determined in the direction of the main, lobar bronchi, trachea.

One of the tasks of MSCT in lung cancer is to determine the boundaries of tumor infiltration and its prevalence in the proximal TBS, which is essential for the planning of the operation. This is due to the close connection in the area of the gates of the lungs and bronchi, large arterial and venous vessels, lymph nodes, and fibrous changes as a result of previous inflammatory processes, which make it difficult to detect tumor infiltration of the main bronchi and trachea according to native CT; however, it is essential for the planning of surgery [17]. Data native MSCT are not always enough to fully answer the question of the defeat of the trachea in lung cancer. Tumor infiltration can be observed in both central and peripheral cancer with centralization. Signs of infiltration at fly-through VB main bronchus, the trachea was narrowing of the lumen, no visualization of cartilage structures: bronchi become deformed tubular structure. The area of preserved cartilage structures indicated the edge of tumor infiltration. According to MSCT VB, three options of neoplastic lesions of the trachea with lung cancer were allocated—predominantly paratracheal (two patients), mainly intrabronchial (three patients), and combined form of infiltration (one patient). In the first variant—peritracheal infiltration—the leading technique was the analysis of images of MinIP, which allowed to clarify the data of the primary MSCT. Semiotic signs in the MinIP mode of infiltration of the external part of the trachea by the tumor were local narrowing of the tracheal lumen. The boundary of the infiltrated tissues, as in the case of bronchial lesions, was determined by the place of visualization of cartilaginous rings and the expansion of the tracheal lumen. With mainly intra-tracheal tumor growth, the leading technique for determining the macrostructure and the lesion boundary was VB and images in MinIP and MIP mode. When this cartilage structure was not visualized, the lumen bumpy, polyp-like mass. Cartilaginous structures of the affected area were not visualized (**Figure 6a–c**).

3D reconstructions in the mode of semitransparent or shaded surfaces were auxiliary in nature, giving a volumetric representation of the extent of changes and supplementing the data of both methods, both in the presence of changes and the boundaries of infiltrative changes. Construction of 3D reconstructions made it possible to obtain a three-dimensional image of the pathology zone and surrounding tissues, including vessels, comparing them with the tumor array, which allows for virtual reconstruction of the surgical intervention zone for optimal choice of surgical tactics.

In five patients, metastatic lesions of the lungs and lymph nodes of the organ gate were revealed (primary kidney cancer in three and colon cancer in two patients). Part of the foci infiltrated segmental, lobar bronchi, enlarged lymph node packages caused their compression, which led to a violation of ventilation of the affected segments and lung lobes up to the development of atelectasis. In VB fly-through of affected bronchi, narrowing lumen nodules and changes in the macrostructure of the bronchial wall in the infiltration zone were clearly identified as secondary foci when compared with the results of the analysis of MinIP images of the zone of interest and data of the native MSCT. When compression of the bronchus of the affected package metastatic lymph nodes were detected luminal narrowing without signs of the wall infiltration (**Figure** 7).

The MSCT data of 17 patients with benign tracheal formations (adenoma, polyp, and others) were analyzed. Benign tumors were characterized by the correct form, a smooth surface, a homogeneous internal structure, the absence of infiltration of the wall, and destruction of the cartilage of the bronchial wall. The localization in the mucous membrane of the tumor was visualized in the lumen of the bronchus, causing narrowing (**Figure 8**).

Papillomatosis, polyps manifested by the visualization of smooth, on the peduncle, the correct form of the structures emanating from the bronchial

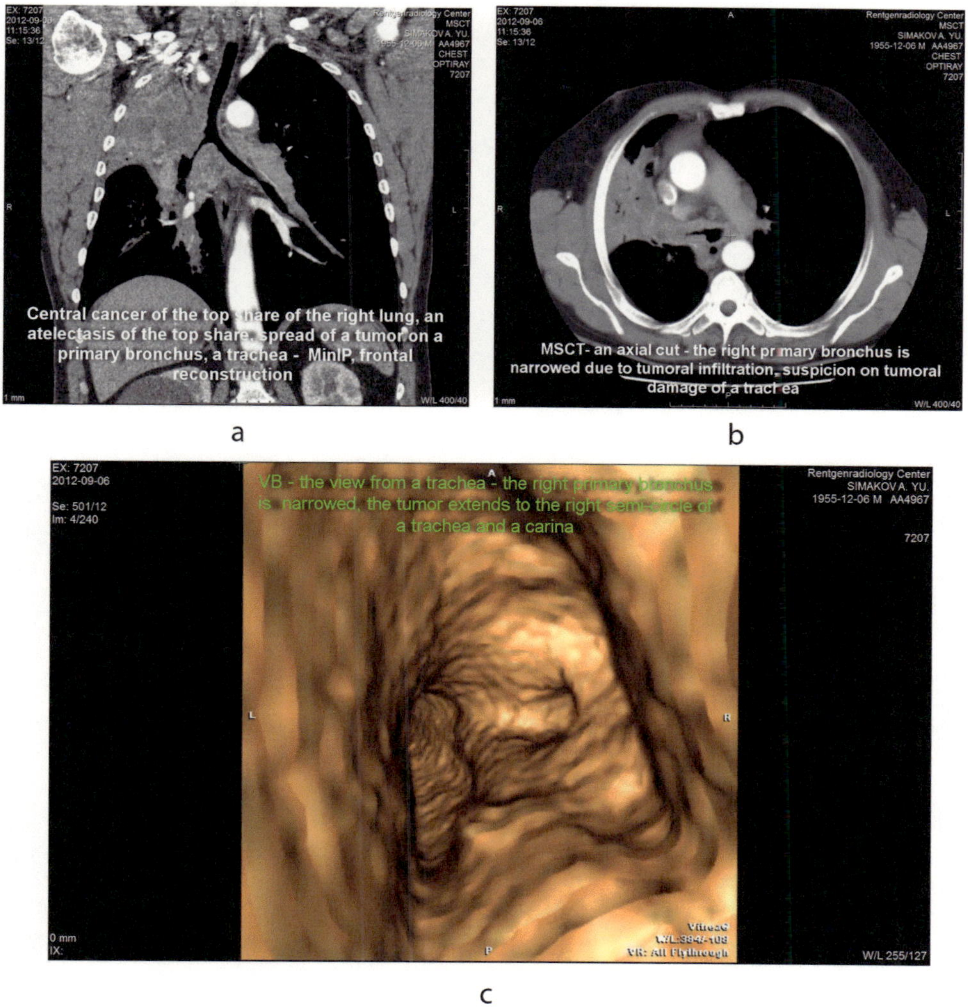

Figure 6.
a. Central cancer of the top share of the right lung, an atelectasis of the top share, spread of a tumor on a primary bronchus, a trachea – MinIP, frontal reconstruction. b. MSCT – an axial cut – the right primary bronchus is narrowed due to tumoral infiltration, suspicion on tumoral damage of a trachea. c. VB – the view from a trachea – the right primary bronchus is narrowed, the tumor extends to the right semi-circle of a trachea and a carina.

mucosa. In some cases, the external pressure of the adjacent single enlarged lymph node can simulate a benign tumor (four patients). Comprehensive data analysis of native MSCT and fly-through VB allowed to determine that the deformation and narrowing of the lumen of the bronchus was associated with the presence of external pressure adjacent to the bronchial lymph node (**Figure 9**). The presence of visual information made it possible to develop a "road map" to perform FBS in order to determine the optimal place for the collection of material for cytological examination, to calculate the depth of the puncture of the wall of the affected bronchus part.

As shown by the combined analysis of native MSCT data and VB techniques, this approach is highly effective in predictive testing of the nature of both primary and secondary TBS lesions. In benign formations (adenoma, polyp, and others), the macrostructure of cartilage structures was preserved, and there was no infiltration of the surrounding tissues. The benign one was protruded into the lumen of the trachea and had the right shape, smooth surface, and homogeneous structure.

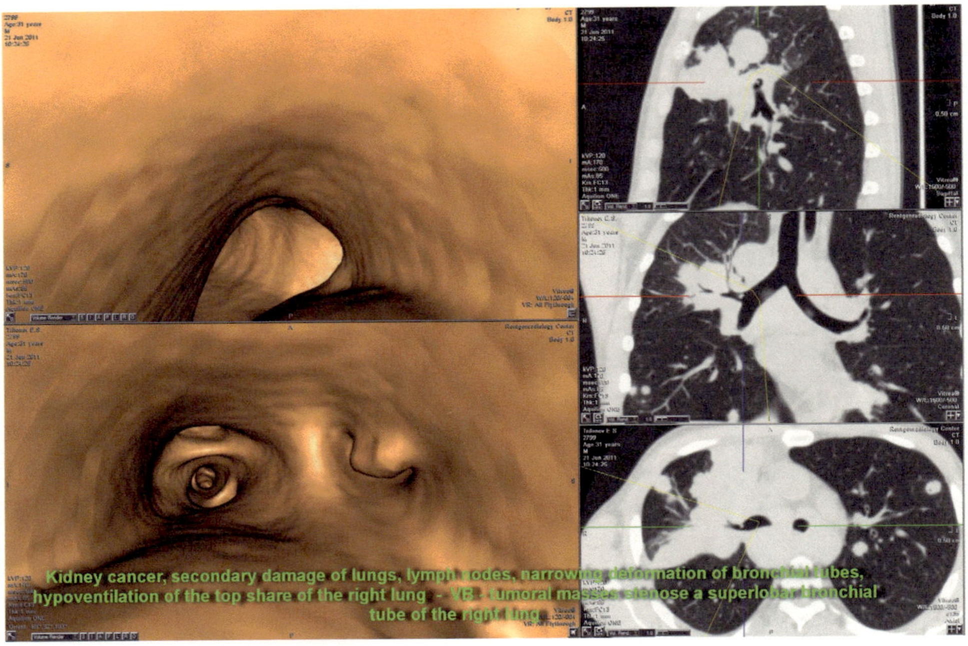

Figure 7.
Kidney cancer, secondary damage of lungs, lymph nodes, narrowing deformation of bronchial tubes, hypoventilation of the top share of the right lung – VB – tumoral masses stenose a superlobar bronchial tube of the right lung.

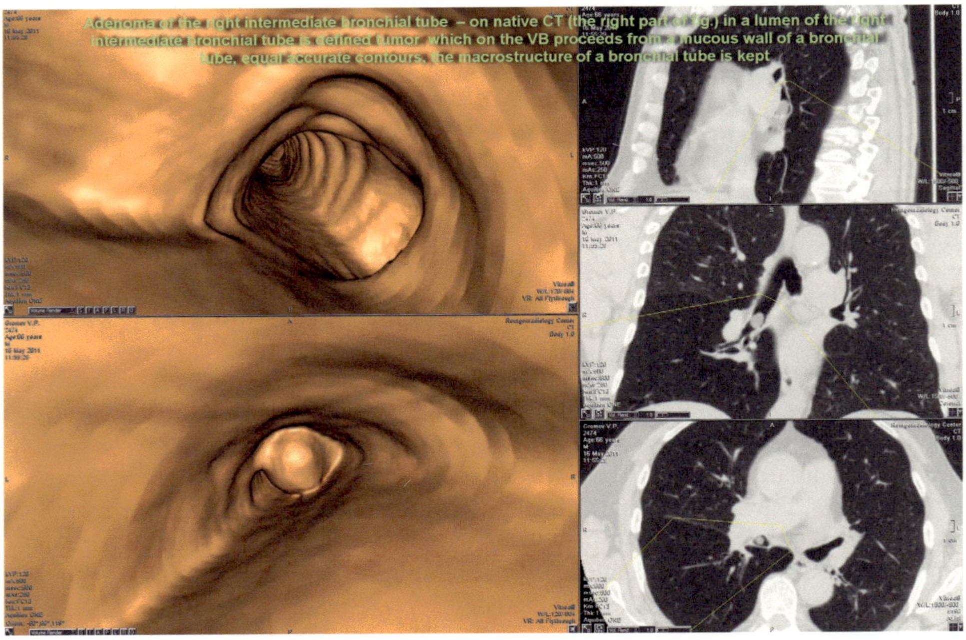

Figure 8.
Adenoma of the right intermediate bronchial tube – on native CT (the right part of fig.) in a lumen of the right intermediate bronchial tube is defined tumor which on the VB proceeds from a mucous wall of a bronchial tube, equal accurate contours, the macrostructure of a bronchial tube is kept.

Malignant lesions were characterized by the presence in the lumen of lumpy tumor masses and the disappearance of the annular structure due to the destruction of cartilage. Peribronchial, paratracheal growth was determined by the narrowing of the lumen with the disappearance of the ring-shaped cartilaginous structures.

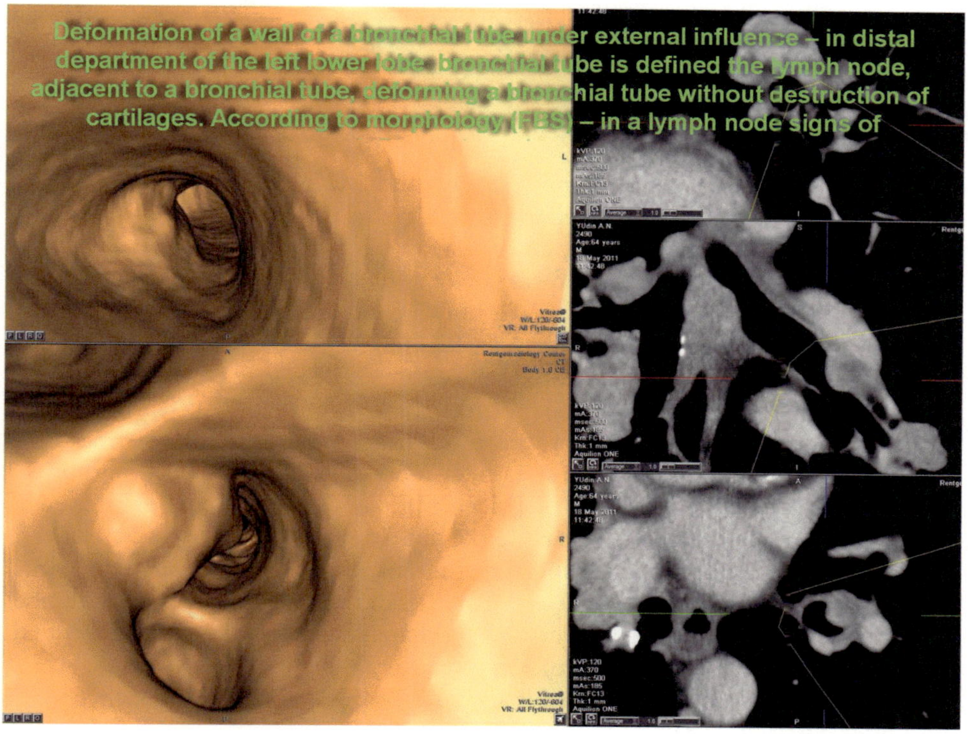

Figure 9.
Deformation of a wall of a bronchial tube under external influence – in distal department of the left lower lobe bronchial tube is defined the lymph node, adjacent to a bronchial tube, deforming a bronchial tube without destruction of cartilages. According to morphology (FBS) – in a lymph node signs of.

1.4 Discussion

The study showed that complex analysis of VB, post-processing images, and native MSCT data allowed obtaining additional information about TBS in lung cancer, secondary lesions, and benign tumors. In contrast to the previous studies, when only the method of VB fly-through was used, it does not allow to agree with the opinion of the authors about the limited possibilities of VB in lung pathology [9, 10]. Most of the studies on VB are based on individual clinical observations and literature data [10, 11, 14, 15]. Our study was conducted on the basis of the analysis of significant clinical material with the development of semiotic signs of TBS lesions and assessment of the diagnostic value of VB methods of their combined analysis with the results of native MSCT. Overall, our opinion about the necessity of wide application in clinical practice CT VB coincides with the result of the work appeared in recent years [11, 13, 15].

1.5 Conclusion

Virtual bronchoscopy of multispiral computed tomography has the possibilities of multiplanar and volumetric reconstructions, post-processing image processing optimal method of diagnosis, determining the probable nature of tumor lesions of the trachea, the prevalence of the process, both outside the body and secondary invasions. In some cases, in stenotic lesions of the trachea, MSCT VB becomes the method of choice in assessing the prevalence of the process. Virtual modeling of intraluminal tracheal tumor, with the data about the surrounding tissues, provides valuable information for the planning of radical treatment.

2. Virtual bronchoscopy multislice computer tomography at traumatic damage of a primary bronchus

2.1 Introduction

Injuries of main bronchi (MB) result from traumatic injury of lungs, as a rule, are combined with injuries of bones of a thorax area. The full separation MB rather rare complication at a thorax injury can be met in 1–3% of cases. In 80% of patients, the rupture comes at the level of bifurcation of a trachea or within 4–2.5 cm from bifurcation of a trachea. Ruptures of MB tubes are met more often on the right. Depending on the severity of the injury, various degrees of damage to the main bronchus are observed—from a small tear to a complete rupture with a divergence of its fragments (partial or complete rupture) are observed [18–20]. The most common clinical manifestations of rupture are chest pain and cough, often accompanied by hemoptysis, shortness of breath, cyanosis due to intense pneumothorax with lung collapse and mediastinal displacement, possible presence of emphysema of the soft tissues of the chest wall and in the neck, and retraction of intercostal spaces. In complicated cases, the presence of intense mediastinal emphysema with extrapericardial cardiac tamponade is noted [21]. Existence or absence of pneumothorax and emphysema generally depends on character and localization of a wound MB. In cases of intrapleural ruptures of the primary and lobar bronchi, there is a tension pneumothorax. At a rupture of a primary bronchus, the lung is switched off from function of breath [22].

Diagnosis of traumatic damages of MB in patients with a thorax injury is a task of tactics of patient treatment; prevention of heavy complications depends on early identification of a rupture of bronchial tubes and a trachea [23]. A MSCT with intravenous administration of a contrast agent the leading noninvasive diagnostic method of consequences of blunt injury of thorax, including their traumatic damage (separation) of a bronchial tube [24–26]. In available literature, studies about the role of the VB of MSCT at traumatic injuries of MB are not found.

2.2 Materials and methods of the research

Data of the VB of MSCT of 10 patients with traumatic injuries of MB as a result of the combined injuries of a thorax—falling from height—3 patients, car accidents—4 patients, and motorcycle—2 patients were analyzed. All patients were brought to the clinic of institute for carrying out reconstructive operations on a primary bronchus from ambulance where they were brought directly after a trauma and received primary medical care and anti-shock therapy.

In seven patients, the rupture was right, and in three, left MB took place (RMB; LMB). The closed pneumothorax took place in eight and opened in two patients. At physical checkup, the expressed dyspnea amplifying at loading, percussion - obtusion of a pulmonary sound, lack of breath. When conducting pneumoscintigraphy with TC-99 m-Makrotekh, a decrease in the size of the lung reduced diffuse inhomogeneous accumulation of the radiotracer at the affected side. The total function of the affected lung was 17–21% and left 82–87%; the difference was 65–66% and violation of 3–4 violation stage capillary blood flow. Capillary blood flow in the intact lung was not disturbed. Traumatic rupture of the MB in all patients is accompanied by fractures of the ribs with displacement on the side of the lesion and hemopneumothorax. All patients underwent reconstructive surgery-isolated resection of the damaged main bronchus with the imposition of tracheobronchial anastomosis. CT with bolus gain of 80–100 ml of the radiopaque medium was carried out on AquilionONE CT scanner (320-slice). Data of native MSCT were supplemented with 3D-volume, multiplanar reconstruction, MinIP mode, and the VB of fly-through at the earlier described technique [4–6, 26]. Controls were carried out in 14–15 days after the transfer from resuscitation to chamber and 40 and more days after operation. Data of the VB of fly-through were compared with results of a bronchofibroscopy (BFS).

2.3 Results of the research

Native MSCT revealed a collapsed lung and a stump MB was defined. Shift of a mediastinum towards the injured lung and existence in a pleural cavity of nonuniform liquid content (with a density up to 45 HU) were noted. The break of MB was defined at distance of 4–30 mm from bifurcation of a trachea—at this length below a carina, the stump of MB tied from tracheas, distal lumen MB, and lobar and segmental bronchi were not visualized. There was hemo, pheumothorax, fractures of ribs, a humeral bone, in 3 - hypodermic emphysema. MSCT with contrast enhancement—the vascular peduncle of the affected lung was safe (**Figure 10**). VB fly-through in all patients revealed various localization break of a primary bronchus through which the pleural cavity with the collapsed lung and existence of level of liquid in a hemithorax were seen. In the area of a rupture, all patients had an uneven bronchial tube stump perimeter because of the "fragmentary" nature of damage (**Figure 11a, b**).

At survey of a trachea, a carina, a contralateral MB, and its branching of data for pathological changes were not revealed. According to FBS data localization, the extent and the nature of the line of a rupture of MB coincided with results of the VB (**Figure 11c**). 3D volume, multiplanar reconstruction, and the image of TBS in MinIP mode significantly supplemented the localizations given by MSCT and VB fly-through in identification, prevalence of traumatic damages, and planning of operation.

Thus, a complex of techniques of the MSCT and VB allowed giving full information about a condition of a trachea, macrostructural changes of the injured MB, and secondary complications of a lung, to receive virtual model of a zone of interest for planning of an operation. Data of MSCT with contrast enhancement and

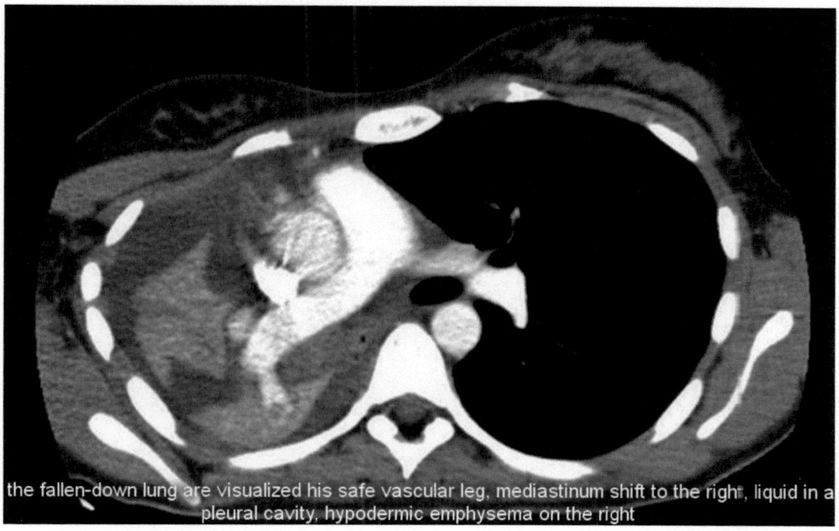

Figure 10.
The fallen-down lung are visualized his safe vascular leg, mediastinum shift to the right, liquid in a pleural cavity, hypodermic emphysema on the right.

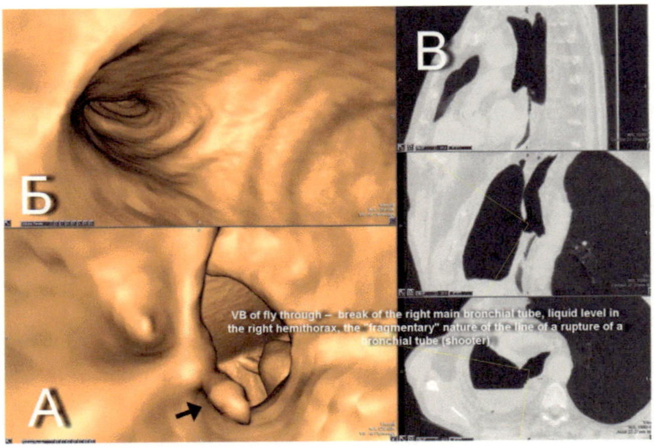

a

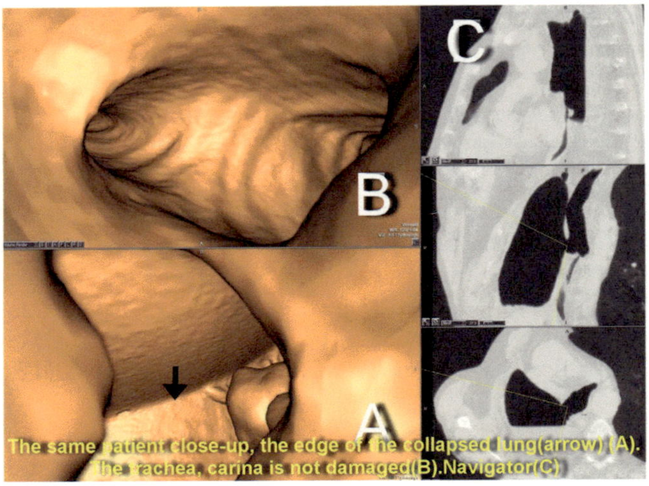

b

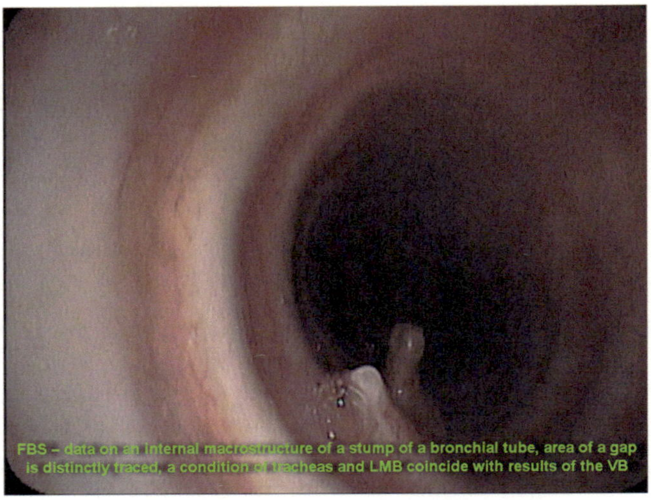

c

Figure 11.
a. VB of fly-through – break of the right main bronchial tube, liquid level in the right hemithorax, the "fragmentary" nature of the line of a rupture of a bronchial tube (shooter). b. The same patient close-up, the edge of the collapsed lung (arrow) (A). The trachea, carina is not damaged (B). Navigator (C). c. FBS – data on an internal macrosturcture of a stump of a bronchial tube, area of a gap is distinctly traced, a condition of tracheas and LMB coincide with results of the VB.

multiplanar reconstruction specified a condition of a vascular lung peduncle on the party of defeat, a complication from a bone skeleton of a thorax, availability of liquid in a pleural cavity, and pneumothorax options.

In 14–20 days after surgical treatment patient control MSCT at an operated lung was carried out; a small amount of air was found in a pleural cavity. At MSCT, it was defined that the lumen of the reconstructed MB was shortened, narrowed, and deformed in the area of an anastomosis. Air filling the lung, MB, and segmental bronchi was restored, the lung completely filling hemithorax. The lumen of the reconstructed bronchial tube was narrowed in the area of reconstruction (**Figure 12**).

MSCT control in four and more months after operation in all patients revealed that the lung was completely normalized, and air and liquid in a pleural cavity were absent. The VB stated restoration of a lumen of a main bronchus with existence of deformation of a lumen in the area of an anastomosis. Similar data on a macrostructure of a zone of an anastomosis were obtained at FBS (**Figure 13a, b**).

2.4 Discussion

As shown, the conducted research of the VB of MSCT gives the chance of a visual estimation of a macrostructure of area of a posttraumatic rupture of MB and assessment of a condition of a trachea and bronchial tubes of a contralateral lung. The comparison of data of FBS and VB showed their full identity in visualization of anatomy of an internal surface of TBS that allows in believing that the VB of MSCT can be a method of choice in monitoring of dynamics of post-operational changes of the reconstructed MB. Combined analysis of the reconstruction of native CT and 3D images in MinIP mode allows studying also an external wall of a bronchial tube that is inaccessible to FBS. VB allows creating a virtual model of area of reconstructive intervention that plays an important role in its planning. As we noted in the introduction, studies on VB traumatic damage to the main bronchi of the lung us were not found in available literature (except the clinical observation published by us) [27, 28].

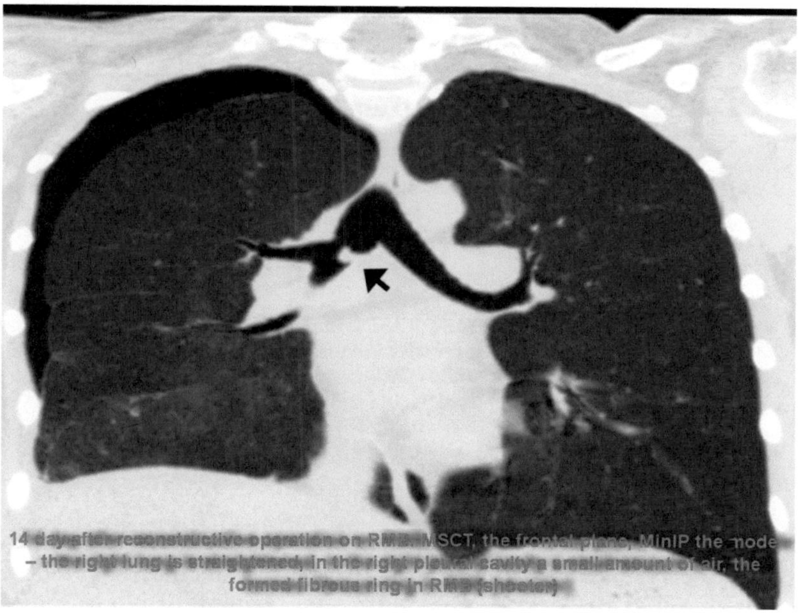

Figure 12.
14 day after reconstructive operation on RMB. MSCT, the frontal plane, MinIP the mode – the right lung is straightened, in the right pleural cavity a small amount of air, the formed fibrous ring in RMB (shooter).

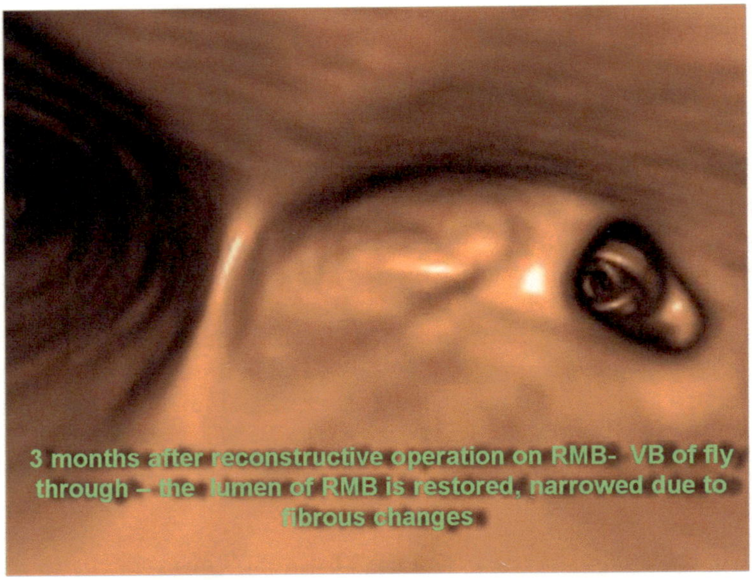

a

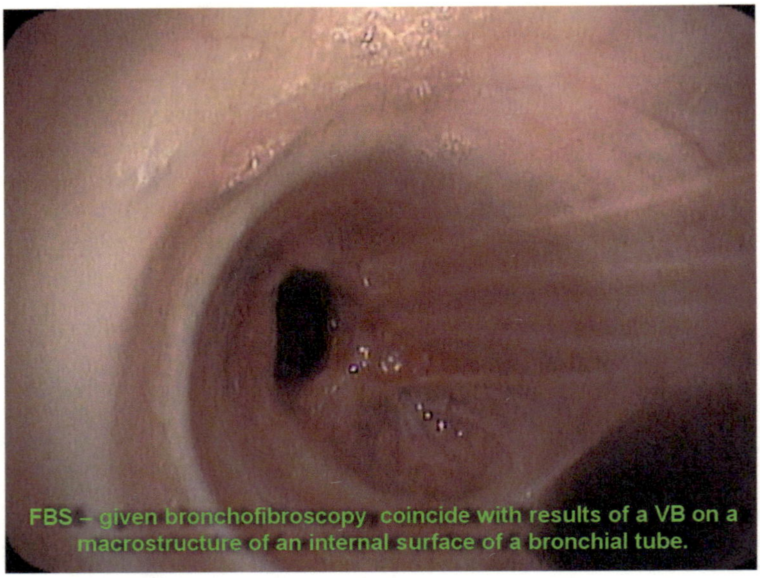

b

Figure 13.
a. 3 months after reconstructive operation on RMB – VB of fly-through – the lumen of RMB is restored, narrowed due to fibrous changes. b. FBS – given bronchofibroscopy coincide with results of a VB on a macrostructure of an internal surface of a bronchial tube.

2.5 Conclusion

At traumatic damages of TBS techniques of the VB MSCT allow to define damages of primary bronchi with high precision, to carry out monitoring of efficiency of reconstructive operations. The combined analysis of multiplanar reconstruction, post-processing, 3D images, and the VB of fly-through allows estimating both internal and external walls of a bronchial tube, to receive the virtual image of reconstructive intervention zone.

Acknowledgements

I would like to express my deep gratitude to Chernichenko Natalia Vasilievna MD, Scientific Research Department of Surgery and Surgical Technologies in Oncology, Russian Scientific Center of Roengenordiology (RSCRR), Moscow, an endoscopist and a specialist in the field of diseases of the chest and abdominal cavity for cooperation.

Conflict of interest

The author declares no conflict of interest and sponsorship when performing this work. The work was performed within the scientific subject of RSCRR Russian Ministry of Health.

Author details

Kotlyarov Peter Mikhaylovich
Research Department of New Technologies and Semiotics Beam Diagnostics of Diseases of Organs and Systems of Russian Scientific Center of Roengenordiology (RSCRR), Moscow, Russian Federation

*Address all correspondence to: marnad@list.ru

References

[1] Malignant neoplasms Russia in 2014. edited by Kaprin AD, StarostinVV, Petrova GVM. 2016. p. 250. (Злокачественныеновобразования России в 2014г. под ред. Каприна АД. Старостина ВВ, Петровой ГВМ. 2016. С.250)

[2] Jugpal TS, Garg A, Sethi GR, et al. Multi-detector computed tomography imaging of large airway pathology: A pictorial review. World Journal of Radiology. 2015;**7**(12):459-474. In Russian

[3] Debnath J, George RA, Satija L, et al. Virtual bronchoscopy in the era of multi-detector computed tomography: Is there any reality? Medical Journal Armed Forces India. 2013;**69**(3):305-310

[4] Kotlyarov P. Temirhanov Z, Flerov E. et al. Virtual bronchoscopy in the diagnosis of lung cancer and its prevalence, monitoring of postoperative changes. Bulletin RSCRR Ministry of Health of Russia. 2013. (URL: http://vestnik.rncrr.ru/vestnik/v13/papers/flerov_v13.htm). In Russian. (Котляров ПМ, Темирханов СЗ, Флеров КЕидр. Виртуальная бронхоскопия в диагностике рака легкого и его распространенности, мониторинге послеоперационных изменений. Вестник РНЦРР. 2013. (URL: http://vestnik.rncrr.ru/vestnik/v13/papers/flerov_v13.htm))

[5] Kotlyarov PM, Temirkhanov ZS, Serbahina EV. Multiplanarr econstruction and virtualbronchoscopyin the evaluation of the statetracheo – bronchial system according Multidetector computed tomography. Radiation Diagnostics and Therapy. 2011. No.2. (2) pp. 50-55. In Russian. (Котляров ПМ, Темирханов ЗС, Щербахина ЕВ. Мультипланарные реконструкции и виртуальная бронхоскопия в оценке состояния трахео – бронхиальной системы по данным мультисрезовой компьютерной томографии. Лучевая диагностика и терапия. 2011. №2. (2) С. 50-55)

[6] Kotlyarov PM, Nudnov NV, Egorova EV. Multidetector computed tomography virtual bronchoscopy in bronchiectasis and osteochondroplasty of bronchopathy. Pulmonology. 2014, No. 4. pp. 68-72. In Russian. (Котляров ПМ, Нуднов НВ, Егорова ЕВ. Мультиспиральная компьютерно–томографическая виртуальная бронхоскопия при бронхоэктатической болезни и остеохондропластической бронхопатии. Пульмонология, 2014, № 4, С. 68-72)

[7] Sdvizcov AM, Yudin AL, Kozhanov LG et al. Multislice computed tomographywith three-dimensional modeling indiagnosing and treatingcancer patients. Bulletin of Moscowcancer Society. 2009. No. 3. pp. 1-4. In Russian. (Сдвижков АМ, Юдин АЛ, Кожанов ЛГидр. Мультиспиральная компьютерная томография с трехмерным моделированием в диагностике и лечении онкологических больных. Вестник Московского онкологического общества. 2009. № 3. С. 1-4)

[8] Adamczyk M, Tomaszewski G, Naumczyk P, et al. Usefulness of computed tomography virtualbronchoscopy in the evaluation of bronchi divisions. Polish Journal of Radiology. 2013;**78**(1):30-41

[9] Aliannejad R. Comment on "Comparison of virtualbronchoscopy to fiber-optic bronchoscopy for assessment of inhalation injury severity". Burns. 2015;**41**(7):1613-1615

[10] Bauer TL, Steiner KV. Virtual bronchoscopy: clinical applications and limitations. Surgical Oncology Clinics of North America. 2007;**16**(2):323-328

[11] Das KM, Lababidi H, Al Dandan S, et al. Computed tomography virtualbronchoscopy: Normal variants, pitfalls, and spectrum of common and rare pathology. Canadian Association of Radiologists Journal. 2015;**66**(1):58-70

[12] Gutiérrez R, Rodríguez SD, Ros Lucas JA. Torsion of middle lobe after lobectomy. correlation between optical bronchoscopy-computed tomography virtual bronchoscopy. Archivos de Bronconeumología. 2015;**51**(7):355-359

[13] Hussein SR. Role of virtualbronchoscopy in the evaluation of bronchial lesions: A pictorial essay. Current Problems in Diagnostic Radiology. 2013;**42**(2):33-39

[14] Luo M, Duan C, Qiu J, et al. Diagnostic value of multidetector CT and its multiplanar reformation, volume rendering and virtual bronchoscopy postprocessing techniques for primary trachea and main bronchus tumors. PLoS One. 2015;**10**(9):e0137329

[15] Osiri X, Sano A, Tsuchiya TJ. Virtual bronchoscopy using OsiriX. Journal of Bronchology and Interventional Pulmonology. 2014;**21**(2):113-116

[16] Terzibaşioğlu E, Dursun M, Güven K et al. The diagnostic efficiency of multislice CT virtual bronchoscopy in detecting endobronchial tumors. Tuberk Toraks

[17] Kharchenko VP, Gvarishvili AA, Eltishev N et al. Examination and treatment of patients with multiple primary malignant tumors of the respiratory system. Bulletin RSCRR Ministry of Health of Russia. 2004. (URL: http://vestnik.rncrr.ru/vestnik/v3/papers/harch14_v3.htm. In Russian). (Харченко ВП, Гваришвили АА, Елтышев НА и др. Обследование и лечение больных с первично-множественными злокачественными опухолями органов дыхания. Вестник РНЦРР Минздрава России. 2004. (URL: http://vestnik.rncrr.ru/vestnik/v3/papers/harch14_v3.html)

[18] Velly JF, Martigne C, Moreau JM, et al. Post traumatic tracheobronchial lesions. A follow-up study of 47 cases. European Journal of Cardio-Thoracic Surgery. 1991;**5**(7):352-355

[19] Scognamiglio G, Solli P, Benni M, et al. Less is more: lung-sparing direct repair of a traumatic rupture of the bronchus intermedius. Journal of Visualized Surgery. 2017;**3**:109. DOI: 10.21037/jovs.2017.06.07. e Collection 2017

[20] Karmy-Jones R, Wood DE. Traumatic injury to the trachea and bronchus. Thoracic Surgery Clinics. 2007;**17**:35-46. DOI: 10.1016/j.thorsurg.2007.03.005

[21] Krawczyk L, Byrczek TP, Łuczyk AM, et al. Traumatic tension pneumopericardium and amputation of the left main bronchus. Polish Journal of Cardio-Thoracic Surgery. 2017;**1**(1):63-65. DOI: 10.5114/kitp.2017.66935

[22] Nishiumi N, Inokuchi S, Oiwa K, et al. Diagnosis and treatment of deep pulmonary laceration with intrathoracic hemorrhage from blunt trauma. The Annals of Thoracic Surgery. 2010;**9**:232-238. DOI: 10.1016/j.athoracsur.2009.09.041

[23] Kummer C, Netto FS, Rizoli S, et al. A review of traumatic airway injuries: potential implications for airway assessment and management. Injury. 2007;**38**:27-33. DOI: 10.1016/j.injury

[24] Kotlyarov PM. Multislice computed tomography: A new stage of development of radiodiagnostics of diseases of the lungs. Medical Imaging. 2011. No. 4. pp. 14-20. In Russian. (Котляров ПМ, Мультисрезовая КТ. новый этап развития лучевой диагностики заболеваний легких. Медицинская визуализация. 2011. №4. С. 14-20)

[25] Cui Y, Ma D-q, Liu W-h. Value of multiplanar reconstruction in MSCT in demonstrating the relationship between solitary pulmonary nodule and bronchus. Clinical Imaging. 2009;**33**:15-21

[26] Kotlyarov PM. Virtual bronchoscopy in the diagnosis of lung cancer. Radiation Diagnosis and Therapy. 2015. № 1. pp. 56-63. In Russian. (Котляров ПМ. Виртуальная бронхоскопия в диагностике рака легкого. Лучевая диагностика и терапия. 2015. № 1. С. 56-63)

[27] Kharchenko VP, Kotlyarov PM, Vinikovetskaya AV et al. Trauma of the right main bronchus (clinical observation). Medical Imaging. 2011. N 4. pp. 76-81. In Russian. (Харченко ВП, Котляров ПМ, Виниковецкая АВ и др. Травматический отрыв правого главного бронха (клиническое наблюдение). Медицинская визуализация. 2011. N 4. С. 76-81)

[28] Kotlyarov PM, Chernichenko NV. Virtual bronchoscopy multislice tomography in traumatic injuries of the main bronchi. Journal of Medical Imaging and Case Reports. 2018. Proceedings of the First International Conference on Medical Imaging and Case Reports (MICR-2018);**2**(2):S25-S26. DOI: 10.17756/micr.2018-suppl 1

Section 3

Pulmonary Hypertention

Chapter 5

Pulmonary Vascular Reserve and Aerobic Exercise Capacity

Vitalie Faoro and Kevin Forton

Abstract

Pulmonary circulation has long been known to have specific proprieties of recruitment and distention to keep the hemodynamic pressure low even when facing very high blood flow. Aerobic exercise especially at high intensity has the particularity to increase considerably the cardiac output. The ability of the pulmonary circulation to face high blood flow with maintaining low pressures is considered as the pulmonary vascular reserve. Furthermore, high pulmonary vascular reserve has been shown to be characterized by low pulmonary vascular resistance, high pulmonary vascular distensibility, high pulmonary capillary volume, and high lung diffusing capacity allowing for lower ventilation at a same metabolic cost. The pulmonary vascular reserve thus reflects the capacity of the pulmonary circulation, including the capillary network, to adapt to high exercise levels. Interestingly, a high pulmonary vascular reserve is an advantage as it is associated with a superior aerobic exercise capacity (VO_2max). This observation strongly suggests that exercise capacity is modulated by the functional state of the pulmonary circulation. However, why or when pulmonary vascular reserve may be related to a higher aerobic exercise capacity remains incompletely understood. The present chapter will discuss the role of each component of the pulmonary vascular reserve during exercise and develop the factors able to influence the pulmonary vascular reserve in heathy individuals.

Keywords: pulmonary circulation, VO_2max, ventilation, diffusion capacity

1. Introduction

During aerobic exercise, muscular contractions increase oxygen peripheral demand proportionally to exercise intensity until a maximal level or maximal oxygen consumption (VO_2max). VO_2max is widely used as a cardiorespiratory fitness indicator as the capacity of oxygen consumption increases with exercise training with values approaching 80–90 ml/min/kg in endurance athletes vs 20–30 ml/min/kg in healthy sedentary subjects. The oxygen consumption is dependent on the interdependence of the different components of the convectional and diffusional oxygen transport systems from ambient air to the mitochondria. Every transport step is a potential VO_2max determinant: ventilation, pulmonary diffusion, blood oxygen transport (depending on cardiac output and arterial oxygen content), muscular diffusion, and mitochondrial activity. The importance of each contribution step varies under different health or environmental conditions. Nevertheless, one can reasonably assume that cardiac output (Q) is most important at sea level, while at higher altitudes, lung or/and muscle diffusion may become more critical [1, 2].

For many years, exercise physiologists have focused on the left side of the heart and the systemic circulation to explain aerobic exercise performance and limitation. However, more recently, robust and growing studies suggest that the right ventricle (RV) might also be an important determinant of maximal cardiac output and VO_2max [3, 4]. More broadly, the RV-pulmonary circulation unit, including the capillary network, has been identified as a potential factor modulating the aerobic exercise capacity in normoxia [5–8] and in hypoxia [7–10]. Indeed, pulmonary vascular reserve, or the ability of the pulmonary circulation to extend, recruit, and vasodilate to smooth an intravascular pressure increase, is critical in minimizing RV afterload and maximizing peak cardiac output at exercise [5, 6]. To discuss the potential importance of this phenomenon, the role of each physiological component of the RV-pulmonary circulation unit and interactions with gas exchange will be reviewed.

2. Right ventricle

Cardiac output increases with exercise intensity in order to ensure oxygen supply to the working muscles. Since the right and left heart are disposed in a series in the cardiovascular system, it is impossible for one ventricle to generate a blood flow exceeding that of the other. The maximal cardiac output is therefore depending on the "weakest" ventricle's performance. Increases in RV afterload may, thereby, possibly serve to limit overall cardiac output [3]. Additionally, the heart being constrained within a stiff pericardium, congestion in the RV may shift the interventricular septum to the left resulting in left ventricular diastolic volume restriction, further limiting maximal Q. This is observable in specific circumstances such as congestive heart failure or highly trained endurance athletes [3].

The normal right ventricle is a thin-walled flow generator perfectly adapted to face the low-pressure, high-compliant pulmonary circulation [3, 11]. However, RV anatomical and physiological properties are maybe not designed to face dramatical afterload increase at high levels of exercise. As compared to the left ventricle (LV), load increases are greater for the RV during exercise [12], and its contractile reserve may become insufficient for adequate blood supply to peripheral demand [12, 13]. Relative to the LV, the greater load that the RV faces during exercise is dominantly attributed to a larger exercise-induced increase in pulmonary artery pressure (PAP) relative to systemic vascular pressure [3].

Increased PAP during exercise is known to limit exercise capacity in pulmonary hypertension patients through a decreased maximum cardiac output by an overloaded right ventricle [11]. Recently it has also been suggested that the same phenomenon could appear in healthy individuals exercising at high workloads at sea level [5–8] but even more at altitude [7–10].

Invasive or noninvasive studies in healthy subjects described a ceiling level of the mean PAP approximating 40–50 mmHg when exercising at maximal workloads corresponding to the extreme afterload level which the RV can face while maintaining a high cardiac output [6, 14–17]. The RV is thus placed under great stress during intense exercise. This leads to the idea that RV outflow might become a limiting factor when the ventricular work demand is overwhelmed, particularly in cases of extreme cardiac outputs (high intensity exercise, endurance athletes) or increased PAP (pathological or hypoxic conditions). Recently, D'Alto et al. demonstrated that echocardiographic RV systolic function indices (tricuspid annular plane systolic excursion (TAPSE), S′, and TAPSE/PAP) correlate with maximal workload in healthy subjects. This finding illustrates that a higher RV contractility reserve, defined as the difference between peak exercise and rest, is an advantage to reach high exercise levels and suggests a potential role of the RV in exercise capacity limitation [13].

3. Pulmonary circulation

3.1 Pulmonary vascular resistance

Pulmonary circulation opposes resistances to the ejecting RV that can be quantified by the PAP at a given cardiac output [18]. According to Poiseuille's law, applicable for a Newtonian fluid flowing laminarly in a straight cylinder, flow and driving pressure are proportional. This would imply that with unchanged resistance every increase in flow would increase PAP. However, the pulmonary circulation has this specific property to reduce resistances by two possible mechanisms: (1) recruitment, enlistment of previously closed pulmonary capillary [19, 20], and (2) distension, expansion of already filled pulmonary capillaries when pressure increases [21]. It is generally accepted that the initial vascular recruitment at the onset of exercise followed by distension allows for the pulmonary circulation to face a high blood flow with limited increase in pressure and maintaining RV systolic function at minimal energy cost [22]. Indeed, low pressure in the pulmonary circulation is essential to prevent two potential exercise capacity limitation mechanisms: fluid leaking from the capillaries to the interstitial space with subsequent gas exchange alterations and RV outflow and oxygen transport limitation [18, 22].

During exercise, PAP increases along with Q but not always with a one to one ratio [15, 23]. In exercising subjects, the PAP can be measured at different exercise intensities or Q allowing for the calculation of the PAP vs. Q slope, as illustrated in **Figure 1**. The PAP vs. Q slope is a more accurate estimation of pulmonary vascular resistance (PVR) as compared to a single measure at rest [14, 22, 24]. Invasive catheterization and noninvasive stress echocardiography studies showed that pulmonary vascular response to exercise varies considerably from one individual to another, with slopes of mean PAP/Q ranging from 0.5 or 1 mmHg/l/min in young adults to 2.5 mmHg/l/min in elderly [14, 23]. This means that with a 10 l/min exercise-induced Q increase, for example, normal PAP increase would range from 5 to 25 mmHg. This great interindividual variability of pulmonary vascular response

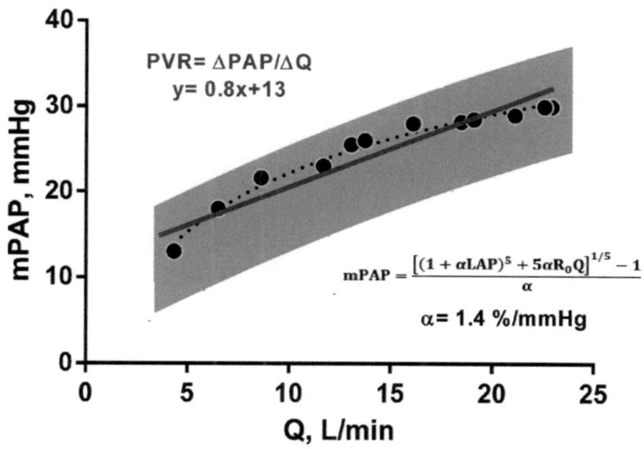

Figure 1.
Stress echocardiography multiple measurements of mean pulmonary arterial pressure (mPAP) at increasing flow (Q) from rest until maximal exercise in one healthy subject. Pulmonary vascular resistance (PVR) is evaluated from the angular coefficient of the mPAP vs. Q linear regression line (ΔmPAP/ΔQ). The PVR of 0.8 mmHg/l/min found in this example is in good agreement with limits of normal (gray background) [23]. From the curvilinearity of this PAP vs. Q relationship (dotted line), a mathematical distensible model relating mPAP, Q, left atrial pressure (LAP), and total PVR at rest (Ro) allows for a calculation of a distensible factor: α (cfr formula). The present subject shows a distensibility (α) corresponding of 1.4% increase of the pulmonary vascular diameter per mmHg of pressure elevation during the entire exercise test and is in good agreement with previous reports [8, 14, 23, 26].

during exercise also suggests a great interindividual variability of RV energy cost. Interestingly, lower PAP/Q slopes have been found in fittest subjects [6–8, 10]. This observation suggests that lower RV output resistance helps to reach higher exercise intensities. Conversely, in patients with pulmonary hypertension, exercise is associated with a sharp increase in PAP (high PAP/Q slopes), and a right ventricular limitation affects exercise capacity [11, 25].

3.2 Pulmonary vascular distensibility

When multiple PAP are measured at increasing exercise or Q levels, it is possible to show that the PAP/Q relationship is not strictly linear but becomes curvilinear with a smoothened pressure increase at higher exercise intensities [14, 16, 26, 27]. The curvilinearity of the PAP/Q relationship reflects the distension of the pulmonary resistive vessels in order to limit the flow-induced pressure increase during exercise. This pulmonary vascular distension participates in decreasing PVR and RV afterload during exercise. The pulmonary vascular distensibility can be quantified with a mathematical model applied to the PA-Q relationship allowing the calculation of a coefficient of distensibility; α (**Figure 1**). Alpha depends on the mechanical properties of the lung vascular walls and represents the percentage change in arteriolar diameter per mmHg of arteriolar pressure increase with exercise [16, 24, 26]. Direct in vitro or indirect in vivo measurements showed an average of 2% increase in diameter per mmHg of distending pressure in healthy pulmonary vessels [14, 26]. Higher alphas, representing a more distensible pulmonary circulation, have been shown to be associated to lower blood flow resistances (PAP/Q slopes) [6]. However, it is interesting to note that the distensibility of the pulmonary vasculature does not stay constant with the onset of exercise but tends to decrease with exercise intensity, indicating that pulmonary vascular compliance decreases along with increases in flow and intravascular distending pressures [6, 16, 23]. Argiento et al. described a mean distensibility α at rest of 2.2%/mmHg decreasing to 1.3%/mmHg at maximal exercise in 88 young heathy adults [23].

Fit subjects, with a high aerobic capacity, have been shown to have enhanced exercise-associated decrease in PVR and increase in pulmonary arterial compliance. This has been demonstrated recently with higher VO_2max correlated to greater pulmonary arteriolar distensibility α [6, 8] associated with lower PVR at maximum exercise or lower PAP/Q slopes [6–8]. This observation was true at sea level but was even more pronounced at moderate or high altitude [7, 8, 10]. One could consider that a more distensible and low resistive pulmonary circulation is an advantage for aerobic exercise performance.

4. Pulmonary capillaries, gas exchange, and ventilation

It has previously been estimated that resistances in the pulmonary circulation are located for 60% at the precapillary level and for 40% at the capillary-venous level [28]. Pulmonary capillaries hemodynamic thus significantly contribute to changes in PVR during exercise and can therefore not be neglected.

4.1 Pulmonary transit of agitated contrast

The property of the pulmonary capillaries to distend during exercise can be studied by intravenous injection of an agitated contrast. Bubbles appearing in the right heart must transit through the pulmonary circulation to be observed in the left heart chambers with echocardiography. At rest, no bubble transit occurs from the right to the left heart. However, during exercise in healthy individuals, pulmonary transit of agitated contrast (PTAC) occurs when contrast appears from the right to the left heart chamber after four to five heartbeats [29, 30]. Whether this exercise-induced bubble transit is explained by pulmonary capillary distension or by the opening of an arteriovenous shunt is still debated [31–33].

In a recent study, La Gerche et al. used PTAC to assess pulmonary vascular reserve in exercising healthy individuals. They observed that subjects with no or minimal bubble transit through the pulmonary circulation also showed higher PVR assessed by steeper PAP/Q slopes, and individuals with high PTAC had lower exercise-induced increases in PAP and greater PVR reduction [5]. This observation suggests that a greater pulmonary vascular reserve can occur through a possible enhanced capillary distensibility. Moreover, this physiological advantage was associated with improved RV function and higher maximal Q. The authors of this study concluded that higher PTAC is advantageous to lower RV afterload and creating less RV fatigue during prolonged and intense exercise [5]. In support of this previous finding, in a similar study, Lalande et al. found that the amount of bubbles transiting through the pulmonary circulation was proportional to the increase in pulmonary capillary pressure and volume during exercise [6]. In this study positive PTAC occurred during exercise when a twofold increase in vascular pressure allowed for a 20–30% increase in capillary blood volume [6]. Capillary recruitment and dilation seem thus crucial to unload the RV at high levels of exercise but is also crucial to maintain capillary pressure low during intense exercise. In numerous studies, West et al. highlighted that an abnormal increase in PAP and subsequent capillary pressure elevation above a 20–25 mmHg threshold at exercise could possibly lead to a capillary stress failure known to elicit interstitial lung edema and altered ventilation/perfusion relationships [34, 35]. Capillary damages have indeed previously been described in some endurance-trained athletes [36].

4.2 Lung diffusion capacity

Capillary blood volume can be estimated noninvasively from lung diffusing capacity measurements using double gas tracers: carbon monoxide (CO) and nitric oxide (NO) differing in their affinity for hemoglobin. The Roughton and Forster equation, $1/DLCO = 1/Dm + 1/\theta Vc$, states that lung diffusion from the alveola to the erythrocyte's hemoglobin is the result of two resistances in series: the alveolo-capillary membrane diffusion component and an intracapillary component. *D*LCO is the measured diffusing capacity of the lung for CO, *D*m the membrane component, θ the hemoglobin affinity for CO, and *V*c the capillary blood volume [37]. Transposing this equation for NO, which has particularly high hemoglobin affinity, two equations can be solved with two unknowns allowing for *V*c calculation [38].

Exercising at sea level is associated with an increase in DLCO, DLNO, Dm, and Vc linearly with the workload intensity without ceiling effect. This suggests that recruitment and distention of the pulmonary circulation does not reach a limit even at high exercise levels. Also, a predominant exercise-induced increase in *V*c relative to *D*m has been described suggesting a predominance of capillary distension rather than recruitment, whereas a recruitment would increase more Dm than Vc [39–41]. This is in keeping with the notion that exercise is associated with an increased diameter of pulmonary capillaries [6, 41–43]. Recent studies found indeed that the amount of blood in the pulmonary capillaries was a determinant of the aerobic exercise capacity [6, 8]. This observation is compatible with the hypothesis that exercise capacity is modulated by the functional state of the pulmonary circulation, including capillary vessels, and could be confirmed in more than 150 healthy adults tested in our laboratory (**Figure 2C**). Additionally, it also appeared that the

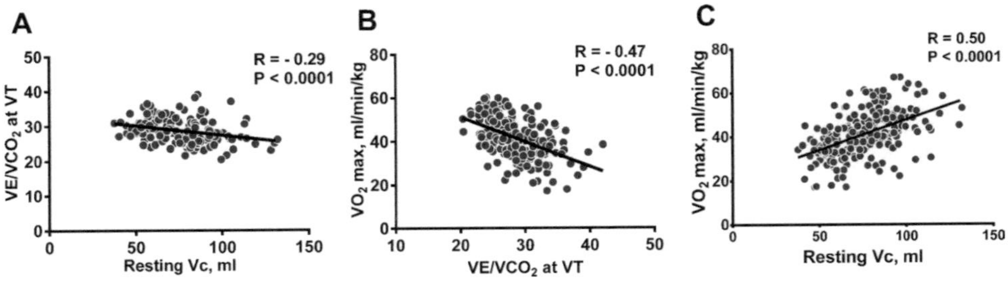

Figure 2.
Correlations between lung capillary volume measured at rest (Vc), ventilatory equivalent for CO_2 (VE/VCO_2) measured at the ventilatory threshold (VT), and aerobic exercise capacity (VO_2max). Larger blood capillary volume allows for better ventilation-perfusion adequacy decreasing ventilation at a given metabolic rate and higher aerobic capacity.

blood volume of the pulmonary capillaries (Vc) measured by the DLCO and DLNO method was correlated to the ventilation at a given metabolic cost (VE/VCO_2 ratio) measured during incremental cardiopulmonary exercise testing (**Figure 2A**). This founding, suggesting that better perfused lungs allows for lower ventilatory cost, is an advantage to reach higher exercise levels (**Figure 2B** and **C**).

The VE/VCO_2 ratio represents the ventilation level needed to evacuate 1 L of CO_2 for 1 minute and is therefore a good indicator of the ventilatory efficiency and represents the metabolic cost of ventilation. The VE/VCO_2 ratio can be measured at the ventilatory threshold, when metabolic acidosis is not yet pronounced and does not substantially influence ventilation. However, the slope of the VE versus VCO_2 relationship from rest until the respiratory compensation point might be more accurate to define the ventilatory chemosensibility [44].

Chronic heart failure and even more so pulmonary arterial hypertension increase the VE/VCO_2 slope by a combination of increased dead space related to low cardiac output, early lactic acidosis, and increased chemosensitivity in the context of an increased sympathetic nervous system tone in relation with the severity of the pathology [45]. The VE/VCO_2 slope has indeed been identified as a strong prognostic tool in patients with heart failure, and in some studies, its prognostic significance has outperformed the VO_2max [44]. In the other hand, endurance athletes are known to have shallow VE/VCO_2 slopes probably through a training-induced decrease in chemosensibility [46].

Interestingly, recent studies also showed a link between higher diffusion capacities (DLNO) and shallowest VE/VCO_2 slopes [6, 8] in keeping with previous notion that higher lung diffusing capacity allows for preserved gas exchange at a lower ventilatory cost [47]. In those studies, the higher diffusion capacities and lower VE/VCO_2 slopes were associated to higher aerobic capacity [6, 8].

5. Pulmonary vascular reserve

The pulmonary vascular reserve is the ability of the pulmonary circulation to accommodate high flows by moderating pressure increase with vascular recruitment, dilatation, and/or distension and allows low hemodynamic pressures in the pulmonary circulation. The more the pulmonary circulation is able to face high blood flow with maintaining low pressures during exercise the greater the pulmonary vascular reserve. This is critical in minimizing RV afterload and maximizing cardiac output during exercise. When pulmonary vascular reserve is compromised, RV ejection may also be compromised, increasing right atrial pressure and limiting maximal cardiac output [18]. Pulmonary vascular reserve avoids abnormal increase in PAP and subsequently increases in pulmonary capillary pressure, protecting from an interstitial pulmonary edema [35, 48]. Finally, a better vascular reserve allows for a greater capillary distention increasing the lung capillary volume which has been shown to be associated with better ventilation-perfusion adequacy, better lung diffusion capacity, and lower ventilatory cost at a given metabolic rate [7, 8].

A pioneer study by La Gerche et al. demonstrated that favorable changes in pulmonary vascular reserve provide a physiological advantage for RV function during exercise [5]. Indeed, subjects with the higher PTAC had the lowest PVR and lowest exercise-induced B-type natriuretic peptide blood levels (usually elevated with ventricular volume and pressure overload) associated with higher maximal Q [5]. Subsequently, Lalande et al. observed that the individuals with the highest VO_2max had the greatest pulmonary vascular reserve, in this study defined as greater arteriolar distensibility α and capillary bed volume along with lowest PVR at maximum exercise [6]. Following these observations, Pavelescu et al. reviewed diffusion capacity measurements and echocardiographic measurements of the pulmonary circulation in a larger number of healthy subjects and confirmed that better aerobic exercise capacity is associated with lower PVR and higher lung diffusing capacity allowing for lower exercise ventilation [7].

Taken together, all those observations strongly suggest that exercise capacity is modulated by the functional state of the pulmonary circulation. A great pulmonary vascular reserve is therefore an advantage in endurance athletic performance especially when exercise is performed at extreme cardiac output levels. However, when or why pulmonary vascular reserve may allow for a higher aerobic exercise capacity is still incompletely described.

6. Influences of pulmonary vascular reserve

It is well-known that interindividual pulmonary vascular response to exercise varies considerably. Beyond that, different factors have been identified to influence the pulmonary vascular reserve such as body position, sex, race, age, and environmental factors.

6.1 Body position

Pulmonary vascular response to exercise testing is either performed in a supine position during catheterization or in a semi-recumbent position during stress echocardiography, while exercise testing is usually performed in a sitting or upright position. Invasive studies previously reported a lower resting PVR in the recumbent position compared with upright position explained by a vascular recruitment when venous return is increased with gravity [49]. However, the authors observed that differences faded and disappeared with exercise-induced cardiac output increase, because of vascular recruitment with pulmonary blood flow elevation. Accordingly, those observations have been confirmed recently by Forton et al. who compared maximal exercise testing in supine, semi-recumbent, and upright positions and showed no body position effect on PAP/Q relationships, alpha, and VO_2max [50].

Influence of posture [17] PAP rest supine (14.0 + −3.3 mmHg) versus upright (13.6 + −3.1 mmHg)

6.2 Race and sex

Racial differences have been suspected to influence pulmonary vascular reserve as black African Americans compared to white Americans of European descent are known to have higher prevalence of hypertension and higher mortality rates for most cardiovascular diseases [51]. Recently, Simaga et al. tested this hypothesis and showed an intrinsically less distensible pulmonary circulation in healthy black sub-Saharan African men as compared to healthy white Caucasians, and this was associated with a lower aerobic exercise capacity [52]. Lower DLNO and DLCO are also reported in Africans as compared to sex-, age-, and body size-matched Caucasians and are explained by racial-related smaller lungs proportionally to body size [53]. However, those racial differences in pulmonary vascular function at exercise did not appear when women were compared [52]. This latest observation is in keeping with previous studies showing that premenopausal women have a more distensible pulmonary circulation with a coefficient of distensibility α up to 45% higher compared to age-matched men [23]. The underlying explanation is not clearly established but might be related to the hormonal context.

6.3 Aging

Exercise capacity decreases with aging, as does the pulmonary vascular reserve. Invasive measurements have previously showed that a reduction in pulmonary microvascular distensibility occurs with age [17, 24]. Consistently, La Gerche et al. noticed that individuals with low PTAC were older than those with positive PTAC [5]. More recently, Argiento et al. confirmed this aging effect observation with noninvasive echocardiographic measurements and showed that while maximal cardiac output was reduced in fifties or older individuals, PAP and PVR were higher with a lower alpha at maximal exercise [23].

Influence of age [17] PAP <30 (12.8 + −3.1 mmHg) versus 30–50 (12.9 + −3.0 mmHg) versus > 50 years (14.7 + −4.0).

6.4 Growth

Aerobic capacity increases gradually with age during childhood and adolescence. The kinetics of this evolution differs in girls and boys related to pubertal hormonal changes reaching a peak in VO_2max earlier in girls compared to boys. However, previous studies showed that VO_2max is not so much a matter of age when VO_2max is corrected by body weight [54, 55].

On the other hand, the maximal workload, endurance time, and maximum average running speed increase continuously with age attesting the complexity of the relations between VO_2 at exercise, weight or body dimensions, and the mechanical performance of muscular work [56].

The progression of endurance time and load at a given VO_2 with age is multifactorial and includes neuromuscular adaptations, movement technique, musculotendinous elastic energy storage, surface vs. weight ratio, body temperature, energy substrates use, and ventilatory response. Indeed, the VE/VCO_2 slope decreases with age reflecting a more efficient ventilatory response during exercise. This has been attributed to chemosensitivity maturation with age [54, 57]. Concomitantly, it is also known that diffusion capacity of DLCO and DLNO increases during adolescence. The link between these two observations remains to be clarified as the DLCO and DLNO increase has previously been mainly attributed to increase in height [58].

Experiments from our exercise laboratory on heathy adolescents show that pulmonary arterial distensibility and chemosensitivity decrease with growth, while maximal Q, RV function and diffusion capacity increase in relation to increased aerobic exercise capacity.

Taken together, the aforementioned findings suggest that the different components of the RV- pulmonary circulation unit are mature at different times. Creating a probable optimal pulmonary vascular reserve and exercise capacity at adulthood but declining further with aging.

6.5 Pollution

Finally, some environmental factors have also been identified as potential pulmonary circulation stressors, namely, altitude and pollution. It has recently been shown that an acute exposure of 2 h to a dilute diesel exhaust increased the pulmonary vasomotor tone by decreasing the distensibility of pulmonary resistive vessels at high cardiac output or high exercise intensities [59]. Further studies are needed for a better understanding of this phenomenon and to evaluate the long-term consequences of diesel exposure on exercise capacity.

6.6 Hypoxia

Increasing visitors and athletes are traveling to altitude but not without consequences on their physical condition. It has long been known that aerobic exercise capacity decreases exponentially with altitude ascent with a significant decline starting above 1000 m. Numerous studies have been conducted in the field, but the underlying mechanisms are until now not fully understood. Although causes might be multifactorial, decreased oxygen transport to the exercising muscle, with a decrease in arterial oxygenation (SpO_2) and an altered maximum Q, is fingered [1, 2, 60].

6.6.1 Right ventricle

At high altitude, in resting conditions, signs of altered diastolic but preserved or enhanced systolic RV function have been described in chronic [61] or acute hypoxic conditions [62, 63]. RV seems thus to tolerate hypoxic conditions. However, a recent study showed inhomogeneous RV contraction in hypoxia but not during exercise, suggesting that hypoxic stress is not trivial [63]. How much this could account for altered RV maximal outflow remains unknown as studies on right ventricular function during hypoxic exercise are sorely lacking [64].

6.6.2 Pulmonary circulation

Since the pioneer study of Von Euler and Liljestrand in 1946 that when airways are exposed to hypoxic air, a local vasoconstrictive reflex modifies the lung perfusion in favor of better oxygenated alveoli [65]. This hypoxic pulmonary vasoconstriction (HPV) is a protective mechanism allowing for substantial improvement in arterial oxygenation [66]. However, at altitude, when the entire lung is hypoxic, a global arteriolar vasoconstriction reduces the pulmonary vascular distensibility and increases the PVR. The subsequent hypoxic pulmonary hypertension is generally mild to moderate [64]. However, during exercise, this substantial increased afterload on the right ventricle might become substantial [64]. Hypoxia may therefore affect the pulmonary vascular reserve with increased likelihood of RV function limitation and/or altered gas exchange by interstitial pulmonary edema or ventilation/perfusion mismatch. How much this accounts for aerobic exercise capacity limitation at high altitude is still a matter of debate.

This last decade, a partial recovery of 10–25% of the hypoxia-induced decrease in maximal oxygen uptake has been reported with intake-specific pulmonary vasodilating interventions [67–72]. Indeed, specific pulmonary vasodilating interventions have been reported to improve the decreased aerobic exercise capacity in hypoxia with little or no effect on normoxic exercise performance. Primary studies described an increase in maximal workload and VO_2max after intake of sildenafil, a phosphodiesterase-5 inhibitor used to treat erectile dysfunction in healthy hypoxic subjects [9, 67–69]. It has been suggested that the underlying mechanism was an increase maximal Q due to a reduced RV afterload after HPV inhibition or pulmonary vasodilation. Similar results were reported after administration of dexamethasone [70] or endothelin receptor blockers [71, 72]. In most of these studies, pulmonary vasodilation effect was also associated with improved arterial oxygenation probably allowing improved oxygen transport to the exercising muscles [69, 73]. De Bisschop et al. showed that pharmacological pulmonary vasodilation improved lung diffusion capacity and also correlated to enhanced exercise capacity at high altitude [74]. The principal suggested underlying mechanisms was related to a pulmonary vasodilation associated decrease in capillary filtration pressure protecting from an interstitial lung edema [74].

6.6.3 Lung diffusion capacity

Acute or chronic hypoxic exposure is associated with enhanced pulmonary diffusion capacity at rest [7, 75, 76]. Moreover, the hypoxia-induced increase in the capillary component being more pronounced than the membrane component suggests a capillary distension in addition to recruitment. This observation has been attributed to increased pulmonary perfusion pressure caused by HPV associated with a venous component of hypoxic vasoconstriction both possibly contributing to increase effective capillary pressure [77].

Interestingly, Taylor et al. showed that recruitment of pulmonary capillaries in response to exercise at high altitude is limited and may therefore be a significant source of exercise limitation [78]. This is keeping with previous correlation found between lung diffusing capacity for nitric oxide (DL_{NO}) and VO_2max at altitude [7, 8, 74].

6.6.4 Pulmonary vascular reserve

The reviewing of data collected during four different high-altitude expeditions (>4350 m) highlighted that individuals with a larger increase in PVR and larger decreased ventilation efficacity with ascent to high altitude were the ones with the greater VO_2max fall [7]. Higher aerobic capacity at high altitude was associated with more pronounced pulmonary vascular reserve as suggested by lower PVR, higher diffusion capacity, and lower VE/VCO_2 [7]. Similarly, pulmonary vascular reserve has been described as an aerobic performance limiting factor in Andean or Himalayan highlanders [10, 79]. This observation has also been confirmed at moderate altitude, even though the overwhelming determinant of decreased VO_2max and maximum workload is a decrease in arterial O_2 content CaO_2 [8].

7. Conclusion

In conclusion, aerobic exercise capacity is depending on the integrity of the different components of the oxygen transfer from ambient air to the mitochondrial cytochromes. The RV function coupling to the pulmonary circulation and the pulmonary capillary network is one of multiple determinants of aerobic exercise capacity. It becomes increasingly clear that a high pulmonary vascular reserve is an advantage for high-intensity exercise performance in heathy subjects. The pulmonary vascular reserve is characterized by lower exercise PAP and PVR and higher pulmonary vascular distensibility associated with greater capillary volume and gas exchange allowing for a lower ventilatory cost at a given metabolic rate. When and how the pulmonary vascular reserve modulates aerobic capacity still need to be clarified. However, age, race, sex, and environmental factors such as pollution and hypoxia have been identified as pulmonary vascular reserve influencers.

Author details

Vitalie Faoro* and Kevin Forton
Cardio-Pulmonary Exercise Laboratory, Université Libre de Bruxelles, Belgium

*Address all correspondence to: vfaoro@ulb.ac.be

References

[1] Wagner PD. New ideas on limitations to VO_2max. Exercise and Sport Sciences Reviews. 2000;**28**(1):10-14

[2] Calbet JA, Boushel R, Radegran G, Sondergaard H, Wagner PD, Saltin B. Determinants of maximal oxygen uptake in severe acute hypoxia. American Journal of Physiology. Regulatory, Integrative and Comparative Physiology. 2003;**284**:R291-R303

[3] La Gerche A, Rakhit DJ, Claessen G. Exercise and the right ventricle: A potential Achilles' heel. Cardiovascular Research. 2017;**113**(12):1499-1508

[4] Stembridge M, Ainslie PN, Shave R. Mechanisms underlying reductions in stroke volume at rest and during exercise at high altitude. European Journal of Sport Science. 2016;**16**(5):577-584

[5] La Gerche A, MacIsaac AI, Burns AT, et al. Pulmonary transit of agitated contrast is associated with enhanced pulmonary vascular reserve and right ventricular function during exercise. Journal of Applied Physiology. 2010;**109**(5):1307-1317

[6] Lalande S, Yerly P, Faoro V, Naeije R. Pulmonary vascular distensibility predicts aerobic capacity in healthy individuals. The Journal of Physiology. 2012;**590**(17):4279

[7] Pavelescu A, Faoro V, Guenard H, de Bisschop C, Martinot JB, Mélot C, et al. Pulmonary vascular reserve and exercise capacity at sea level and at high altitude. High Altitude Medicine and Biology. 2013;**14**(1):19-26

[8] Faoro V, Deboeck G, Vicenzi M, Gaston AF, Simaga B, Doucende G, et al. Pulmonary vascular function and aerobic exercise capacity at moderate altitude. Medicine and Science in Sports and Exercise. 2017;**49**(10):2131-2138

[9] Ghofrani HA, Reichenberger F, Kohstall MG, Mrosek EH, Seeger T, Olschewski H, et al. Sildenafil increased exercise capacity during hypoxia at low altitudes and at Mount Everest Base camp. Annals of Internal Medicine. 2004;**141**:169-177

[10] Faoro V, Huez S, Vanderpool R, Groepenhoff H, de Bisschop C, Martinot JB, et al. Pulmonary circulation and gas exchange at exercise in Sherpas at high altitude. The Journal of Applied Physiology. 2014;**116**(7):919-926

[11] Champion HC, Michelakis ED, Hassoun PM. Comprehensive invasive and noninvasive approach to the right ventricle-pulmonary circulation unit: State of the art and clinical and research implications. Circulation. 2009;**120**:992-1007

[12] La Gerche A, Heidbüchel H, Burns AT, Mooney DJ, Taylor AJ, Pfluger HB, et al. Disproportionate exercise load and remodeling of the athlete's right ventricle. Medicine and Science in Sports and Exercise. 2011;**43**:974-981

[13] D'Alto M, Pavelescu A, Argiento P, Romeo E, Correra A, Di Marco GM, et al. Echocardiographic assessment of right ventricular contractile reserve in healthy subjects. Echocardiography. 2017;**34**(1):61-68

[14] Reeves JT, Dempsey JA, Grover RF. Pulmonary circulation during exercise. In: Weir EK, Reeves JT, editors. Pulmonary Vascular Physiology and Physiopathology. New York, NY: Marcel Dekker; 1989. pp. 107-133

[15] Bossone E, Rubenfire M, Bach DS, Ricciardi M, Armstrong WF. Range of tricuspid regurgitation velocity at rest

and during exercise in normal adult men: Implications for the diagnosis of pulmonary hypertension. Journal of the American College of Cardiology. 1999;**33**:1662-1666

[16] Argiento P, Chesler N, Mule M, D'Alto M, Bossone E, Unger P, et al. Exercise stress echocardiography for the study of the pulmonary circulation. The European Respiratory Journal. 2010;**35**:1273-1278

[17] Kovacs G, Berghold A, Scheidl S, Olschewski H. Pulmonary arterial pressure during rest and exercise in healthy subjects: A systematic review. The European Respiratory Journal. 2009;**34**(4):888-894

[18] Pinsky MR. The right ventricle: Interaction with the pulmonary circulation. Critical Care. 2016;**20**:266

[19] Hanson WL, Emhardt JD, Bartek JP, Latham LP, Checkley LL, Capen RL, et al. Site of recruitment in the pulmonary microcirculation. Journal of Applied Physiology. 1989;**66**:2079-2083

[20] Presson RG Jr, Baumgartner WA Jr, Peterson AJ, Glenny RW, Wagner WW Jr. Pulmonary capillaries are recruited during pulsatile flow. Journal of Applied Physiology. 2002;**92**:1183-1190

[21] Rosenzweig DY, Hughes JM, Glazier JB. Effects of transpulmonary and vascular pressures on pulmonary blood volume in isolated lung. Journal of Applied Physiology. 1970;**28**:553-560

[22] Naeije R, Chesler N. Pulmonary circulation at exercise. Comprehensive Physiology. 2012;**2**(1):711-741

[23] Argiento P, Vanderpool RR, Mule M, et al. Exercise stress echocardiography of the pulmonary circulation: Limits of normal and sex differences. Chest. 2012;**590**:4279-4288

[24] Reeves JT, Linehan JH, Stenmark KR. Distensibility of the normal human lung circulation during exercise. American Journal of Physiology. Lung Cellular and Molecular Physiology. 2005;**288**:L419-L425

[25] Claessen G, La Gerche A, Wielandts JY, Bogaert J, Van Cleemput J, Wuyts W, et al. Exercise pathophysiology and sildenafil effects in chronic thromboembolic pulmonary hypertension. Heart. 2015;**101**(8):637-644

[26] Linehan JH, Haworth ST, Nelin LD, Krenz GS, Dawson CA. A simple distensible vessel model for interpreting pulmonary vascular pressure-flow curves. Journal of Applied Physiology. 1992;**73**:987-994

[27] Krenz GS, Dawson CA. Flow and pressure distributions in vascular networks consisting of distensible vessels. American Journal of Physiology. Heart and Circulatory Physiology. 2003;**284**:H2192-H2203

[28] Cope DK, Grimbert F, Downey JM, Taylor AE. Pulmonary capillary pressure: A review. Critical Care Medicine. 1992;**20**:1043-1056

[29] Eldrige MW, Dempsey JA, Haverkamp HC, Lovering AT, Hokanson JS. Exercise-induced intrapulmonary arteriovenous shunting in healthy humans? Journal of Applied Physiology. 2004:797-805

[30] Stickland MK, Welsh RC, Haykowsky MJ, Petersen SR, Anderson WD, Taylor DA, et al. Intra-pulmonary shunt and pulmonary gas exchange during exercise in humans. The Journal of Physiology. 2004;**561**:321-329

[31] Hopkins SR, Olfert IM, Wagner PD. Point: Exercise-induced intrapulmonary shunting is imaginary. Journal of Applied Physiology. 2009;**107**:993-994

[32] Lovering AT, Eldridge MW, Stickland MK. Counterpoint: Exercise-induced intrapulmonary shunting is real. Journal of Applied Physiology. 2009;**107**:994-997

[33] Naeije R, Faoro V. Pathophysiological insight into shunted bubbles. Journal of Applied Physiology. 2009;**107**(3):999-1000

[34] West JB, Tsukimoto K, Mathieu-Costello O, Prediletto R. Stress failure in pulmonary capillaries. Journal of Applied Physiology (Bethesda Md):1985. 1991;**70**(4):1731-1742

[35] West JB, Mathieu-Costello O. Stress failure of pulmonary capillaries as a limiting factor for maximal exercise. European Journal of Applied Physiology. 1995;**70**(2):99-108

[36] Prefaut C, Durand F, Mucci P, Caillaud C. Exercise-induced arterial hypoxaemia in athletes: A review. Sports medicine (Auckland, N.Z.). 2000;**30**(1):47-61

[37] Roughton FJ, Forster RE. Relative importance of diffusion and chemical reaction rates in determining rate of exchange of gases in the human lung, with special reference to true diffusing capacity of pulmonary membrane and volume of blood in the lung capillaries. Journal of Applied Physiology. 1957;**11**:290-302

[38] Guénard H, Varene N, Vaida P. Determination of lung capillary blood volume and membrane diffusing capacity in man by the measurements of NO and CO transfer. Respiratory Physiology. 1987;**70**:113-120

[39] Johnson RL Jr, Spicer WS, Bishop JM, Forster RE. Pulmonary capillary blood volume, flow and diffusing capacity during exercise. Journal of Applied Physiology. 1960;**15**:893-902

[40] Glenet SN, De Bisschop C, Vargas F, Guénard HJ. Deciphering the nitric oxide to carbon monoxide lung transfer ratio: Physiological implications. The Journal of Physiology. 2007;**582**:767-775

[41] Hsia CC, McBrayer DG, Ramanathan M. Reference values of pulmonary diffusing capacity during exercise by a rebreathing technique. American Journal of Respiratory and Critical Care Medicine. 1995;**152**:658-665

[42] Tamhane RM, Johnson RL Jr, Hsia CC. Pulmonary membrane diffusing capacity and capillary blood volume measured during exercise from nitric oxide uptake. Chest. 2001;**120**(6):1850-1856

[43] Zavorsky GS, Quiron KB, Massarelli PS, Lands LC. The relationship between single-breath diffusion capacity of the lung for nitric oxide and carbon monoxide during various exercise intensities. Chest. 2004;**125**(3):1019-1027

[44] Arena R, Myers J, Aslam SS, Varughese EB, Peberdy MA. Peak VO_2 and VE/VCO_2 slope in patients with heart failure: A prognostic comparison. American Heart Journal. 2004;**147**(2):354-360

[45] Deboeck G, Niset G, Lamotte M, Vachiéry JL, Naeije R. Exercise testing in pulmonary arterial hypertension and in chronic heart failure. The European Respiratory Journal. 2004;**23**(5):747-751

[46] Martin BJ, Sparks KE, Zwillich CW, Weil JV. Low exercise ventilation in endurance athletes. Medicine and Science in Sports. 1979;**11**(2):181-185

[47] Dempsey JA, Reddan WG, Birnbaum ML, Forster HV, Thoden JS, Grover R, et al. Effects of acute through life-long hypoxic exposure on exercise pulmonary gas exchange. Respiration Physiology. 1971;**13**:62-89

[48] West JB. Fragility of pulmonary capillaries. Journal of Applied Physiology. 2013;**115**:1-15

[49] Reeves JT, Taylor AE. Pulmonary hemodynamics and fluid exchange in the lungs at exercise. Handbook of Physiology. 1999; Section 12:585-613

[50] Forton K, Motoji Y, Deboeck G, Faoro V, Naeije R. Effects of body position on exercise capacity and pulmonary vascular pressure-flow relationships. Journal of Applied Physiology. 2016;**121**(5):1145-1150

[51] Jones DW, Hall JE. Racial and ethnic differences in blood pressure. Biology and Sociology. Circulation. 2006;**114**:2757-2759

[52] Simaga B, Vicenzi M, Faoro V, Caravita S, Di Marco G, Forton K, et al. Pulmonary vascular function and exercise capacity in black sub-Saharan Africans. Journal of Applied Physiology. 2015;**119**(5):502-507

[53] Simaga B, Forton K, Motoji Y, Naeije R, Faoro V. Lung diffusing capacity in sub-Saharan Africans versus European Caucasians. Respiratory Physiology and Neurobiology. 2017;**241**:23-27

[54] Ten Harkel AD, Takken T, Van Osch-Gevers M, Helbing W. Normal values for cardiopulmonary exercise testing in children. European Journal of Cardiovascular Prevention and Rehabilitation. 2011;**18**:48-54

[55] Tavares AC, Bocchi EA, Teixeira-Neto IS, Guimarães GV. A meta-analysis of cardiopulmonary exercise testing in pre-pubertal healthy children produces new information. Medical Express. 2016;**3**(1):1-9

[56] Cooper DM, Leu SY, Galassetti P, Radom-Aizik S. Dynamic interactions of gas exchange, body mass, and progressive exercise in children. Medicine and Science in Sports and Exercise. 2014;**46**:877-886

[57] Parazzi P, Marson F, Ribeiro M, Schivinski C, Ribeiro J. Ventilatory efficiency in children and adolescents: A systematic review. Disease Markers. 2015;**1**:1-10

[58] Thomas A, Hanel B, Marott JL, Buchvald F, Mortensen J, et al. The single-breath diffusing capacity of CO and NO in healthy children of European descent. PLoS One. 2014;**9**(12):e113177

[59] Wauters A, Vicenzi M, De Becker B, Riga JP, Esmaeilzadeh F, Faoro V, et al. At high cardiac output, diesel exhaust exposure increases pulmonary vascular resistance and decreases distensibility of pulmonary resistive vessels. American Journal of Physiology. Heart and Circulatory Physiology. 2015;**309**(12):H2137-H2144

[60] Fulco CS, Rock PB, Cymerman A. Maximal and submaximal exercise performance at altitude. Aviation, Space, and Environmental Medicine. 1998;**69**(8):793-801

[61] Huez S, Faoro V, Guénard H, Martinot JB, Naeije R. Echocardiographic and tissue Doppler imaging of cardiac adaptation to high altitude in native highlanders versus acclimatized lowlanders. The American Journal of Cardiology. 2009;**103**:1605-1609

[62] Netzer NC, Strohl KP, Högel J, Gatterer H, Schilz R. Right ventricle dimensions and function in response to acute hypoxia in healthy human subjects. Acta Physiologica. 2017;**219**(2):478-485

[63] Pezzuto B, Forton K, Badagliacca R, Motoji Y, Faoro V, Naeije R. Right ventricular dyssynchrony during hypoxic breathing but not during exercise in healthy subjects: A speckle tracking echocardiography

study. Experimental Physiology. 2018;**103**(10):1338-1346

[64] Naeije R, Dedobbeleer C. Pulmonary hypertension and the right ventricle in hypoxia. Experimental Physiology. 2013;**98**(8):1247-1256

[65] Von Euler US, Liljestrand G. Observations on the pulmonary arterial blood pressure in the cat. Acta Physiologica Scandinavica. 1946;**12**:301-320

[66] Brimioulle S, Julien V, Gust R, Kozlowski JK, Naeije R, Schuster DP. Importance of hypoxic vasoconstriction in maintaining oxygenation during acute lung injury. Critical Care Medicine. 2002;**30**(4):874-880

[67] Richalet JP, Gratadour P, Robach P, Pham I, Dechaux M, Joncquirt-Latarjet A, et al. Sildenafil inhibits altitude-induced hypoxemia and pulmonary hypertension. American Journal of Respiratory and Critical Care Medicine. 2005;**171**:275-281

[68] Hsu AR, Barnholt KE, Grundmann NK, Lin JH, McCullum SW, Friedlander AL. Sildenafil improves cardiac output and exercise performance during acute hypoxia, but not normoxia. Journal of Applied Physiology. 2006, 2006;**100**:2031-2040

[69] Faoro V, Lamotte M, Deboeck G, Pavelescu A, Huez S, Guenard H, et al. Effects of sildenafil on exercise capacity in hypoxic normal subjects. High Altitude Medicine and Biology. 2007;**8**:155-163

[70] Fischler M, Maggiorini M, Dorschner L, Debrunner J, Bernheim A, Kiencke S, et al. Dexamethasone but not tadalafil improves exercise capacity in adults prone to high altitude pulmonary edema. American Journal of Respiratory and Critical Care Medicine. 2009;**180**:346-352

[71] Faoro V, Boldingh S, Moreels M, Martinez S, Lamotte M, Unger P, et al. Bosentan decreases pulmonary vascular resistance and improves exercise capacity in acute hypoxia. Chest. 2009;**135**:1215-1222

[72] Naeije R, Huez S, Lamotte M, Retailleau K, Neupane S, Abramowicz D, et al. Pulmonary artery pressure limits exercise capacity at high altitudes. The European Respiratory Journal. 2010;**36**:1049-1055

[73] Olfert IM, Loeckinger A, Treml B, Faulhaber M, Flatz M, Burtscher M, et al. Sildenafil and bosentan improve arterial oxygenation during acute hypoxic exercise: A controlled laboratory trial. Wilderness and Environmental Medicine. 2011;**22**:211-221

[74] de Bisschop C, Martinot JB, Leurquin-Sterk FV, Guenard H, Naeije R. Improvement in lung diffusion by endothelin a receptor blockade at high altitude. Journal of Applied Physiology. 2011;**112**(1):20-25

[75] Snyder EM, Olson TP, Johnson BD, Frantz RP. Influence of sildenafil on lung diffusion during exposure to acute hypoxia at rest and during exercise in healthy humans. European Journal of Applied Physiology. 2008;**103**(4):421-430

[76] Agostoni P, Swenson ER, Bussotti M, Revera M, Meriggi P, Faini A, et al. High-altitude exposure of three weeks duration increases lung diffusing capacity in humans. Journal of Applied Physiology. 2011;**110**(6):1564-1571

[77] Maggiorini M, Mélot C, Pierre S, Pfeiffer F, Greve I, Sartori C, et al. High altitude pulmonary edema is initially caused by an increased capillary pressure. Circulation. 2001;**103**:2078-2083

[78] Taylor BJ, Coffman KE, Summerfield DT, Issa AN, Kasak AJ, Johnson BD. Pulmonary capillary reserve and exercise capacity at high altitude in healthy humans. European Journal of Applied Physiology. 2016;**116**(2):427-437

[79] Groepenhoff H, Overbeek MJ, Mulè M, van der Plas M, Argiento P, Villafuerte FC, et al. Exercise pathophysiology in patients with chronic mountain sickness exercise in chronic mountain sickness. Chest. 2012;**142**(4):877-884

Chapter 6

2-Methoxyestradiol in Pulmonary Arterial Hypertension: A New Disease Modifier

Stevan P. Tofovic and Edwin K. Jackson

Abstract

Pulmonary arterial hypertension (PAH), a debilitating and incurable disease, predominantly develops in women. Estradiol metabolism leads to the production of numerous metabolites with different levels of estrogenic activity and very often opposing biological effects. Dysregulated estradiol metabolism was recently linked to the penetrance, progression, and prognosis of the disease. Ongoing clinical trials are examining the effects of estradiol synthesis/signaling inhibition in patients with PAH. In this chapter, the effects of sex, sex hormones, and estradiol metabolism on the healthy pulmonary circulation and vascular pathobiology are discussed in the light of estradiol metabolism as potential pharmacological target in PAH. The effects of estrogens and their metabolites on vascular pathobiology and disease progression, their involvement in PAH-associated diseases, and the pros and cons for interventions at different levels of estradiol metabolism are discussed. Finally, we propose that 2-methoxyestradiol (2ME), a major non-estrogenic metabolite of estradiol, mediates at least in part the beneficial effects of estradiol and that 2ME exhibits opposing effects to estradiol on several processes relevant to the underlying pathophysiology of PAH, including angiogenesis, metabolic reprogramming, inflammation, and immunity. Based on cellular and in vivo effects, 2ME should be viewed as a disease modifier in women with PAH.

Keywords: pulmonary hypertension, estradiol metabolism, 2-methoxyestradiol, angiogenesis, inflammation

1. Introduction

Pulmonary arterial hypertension (PAH) is a progressive incurable disease of pulmonary vasculature that ultimately leads to failure of the right ventricle (RV) and death. Notably the disease predominantly develops in women. The first report in 1951 by Dr. David Dresdale and colleagues from Maimonides Hospital of Brooklyn on hemodynamic aspects of primary pulmonary hypertension (PH) included three 25- to 35-year-old women [1]. Similarly, in 1952 in the second seminal report on PAH, British cardiologist Paul Wood recognized that this is "...relatively rare disease, usually encountered in women between 20 and 30, but may be met at any age and in either sex..." [2]. These early observations of female preponderance of PAH were confirmed by epidemiological studies conducted in the last two decades, and the data from various registries worldwide report a female-to-male ratio (F:M) ranging from 2:1 to 4:1 [3–9] and up to 4:1 to 9:1 for connective tissue disease [10–12]. However, with aging the female preponderance of disease disappears, and an M:F of only 1.2:1.0 has been reported in elderly PAH patients [13]. The latter strongly suggests involvement of female sex hormones in the development of PAH.

1.1 Vascular pathobiology in PAH

Pulmonary vascular remodeling is a pathological hallmark of PAH. Vascular morphological manifestations of the disease include (i) concentric and asymmetric obliterative proliferation of endothelial cells (ECs) and distal formation of multicellular plexiform lesions (PLXL); (ii) the muscularization of distal non-musculinized precapillary vessels; (iii) adventitia remodeling in form of fibrosis, inflammation, and perivascular edema; and (iv) PLXL, dilation lesions, and arteritis classified as complex lesions [14]. Three-dimensional analysis of vascular lesions in patients with severe PAH reveals the existence of two major phenotypes of ECs. The normal quiescent apoptosis-sensitive ECs are located in the peripheral areas of the lesion, are negative for phosphorylated MAPK, and have a high expression of p27kip1 (a marker of slow proliferation). The highly proliferative apoptosis-resistant cells in the central core of the vascular lesion have elevated MAPK activity and increased expression of HIF-1α, VEGF protein, and VEGF-2 receptor and low expression of p27kip1 [15, 16].

Both inflammation and immune cell response are recognized as important pathogenic factors in PAH [17–19]. For example, in experimental PH perivascular inflammation, due to macrophages, mast cells, and T and B lymphocytes, precedes vascular remodeling and elevated pulmonary pressure [20], and in PAH patients, the degree of perivascular infiltration by immune cells correlates with vascular remodeling and pulmonary artery pressure [21]. As discussed below, inflammation may markedly influence estradiol metabolism, and vice versa, estrogens and their metabolites may instigate, perpetuate, or inhibit inflammation and modulate immune cell responses in PAH.

2. Opposing effects of estradiol and 2-methoxyestradiol on estrogen metabolism

Since our first report that 2ME, a major non-estrogenic metabolite of 17β-estradiol (E2), attenuates the development and progression of monocrotaline (MCT)-induced PH and that estrogens may be pathogenic in PAH [22], a growing body of evidence suggests the involvement of dysregulated estradiol metabolism and elevated estrogen levels in the development, progression, and prognosis of PAH.

2.1 Increased estradiol production in PAH

Formation and metabolism of estrogens are complex (**Figure 1**). The pivotal precursors for synthesis of both androgens and estrogens are dehydroepiandrosterone (DHEA) and its biologically inactive sulfate (DHEA-S). DHEA is produced in the adrenal gland of men and postmenopausal women and in the ovaries and placenta of premenopausal women. DHEA, the most abundant steroid in circulation, is also produced by peripheral conversion from circulating DHEA-S. DHEA is transported into cells by organic anion transporters (OATPs) that are expressed in various tissues including the endothelial and inflammatory cells and lungs [23–25]. The delicate balance between DHEA and DHEA-S is controlled by the relative activity of sulfotransferase (DHEA → DHEA-S) and sulfatase (DHEA-S → DHEA) [26]. Both DHEA and DHEA-S are protective in experimental models of pulmonary

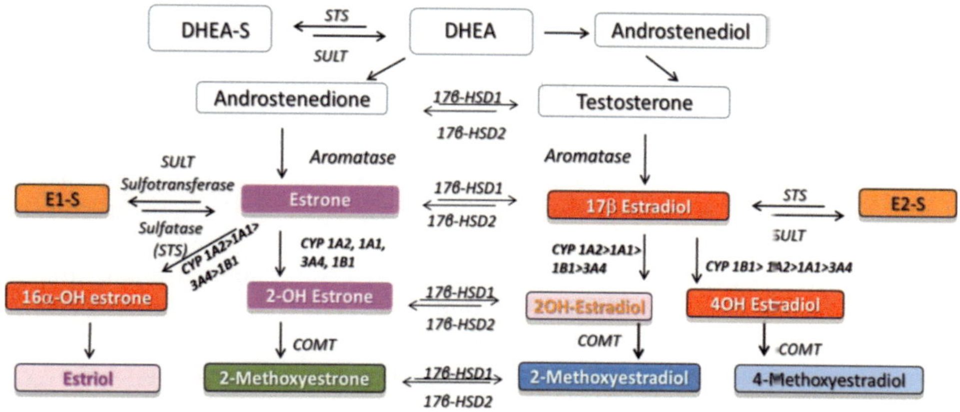

Figure 1.
Dehydroepiandrosterone is the most abundant steroid in circulation that is also produced by peripheral conversion from its circulating inactive sulfated metabolite DHEA-S. The balance between inactive sulfated sex steroids and sex steroids and their biologically active metabolites and metabolic precursors is controlled by sulfatase (STS) and sulfotransferase (SULT). Aromatase is a key enzyme in estrogen production because this enzyme controls aromatization of androgenic precursors to estrogens and intracrine production of estrogens. 2-Hydroxylation/methylation pathway of estrogen metabolism produces non-estrogenic metabolites with opposite effects to maternal estrogens. Hydroxylation of estradiol (E2) at C4 and C16 position leads to production of highly estrogenic metabolites with proliferative, pro-inflammatory, and angiogenic properties.

hypertension [27–31] including models of angioproliferative PH [32, 33]. Recently, lower DHEA-S and higher E2 levels have been linked to a greater risk of PAH and worse hemodynamics, functional status, and greater risk of death [34, 35]. Notably, DHEA improves PAH in patients with obstructive pulmonary disease [36], a finding supporting the potential therapeutic application of DHEA in PAH patients. DHEA is an over-the-counter supplement with no major side effects; however, its safety during chronic use in pharmacological doses is unknown. One potential adverse effect in this regard would be increased circulating/tissue E2 levels that may exacerbate endothelial remodeling and inflammation (infra vide).

Aromatase (encoded by the CYP19A1 gene) is the rate-limiting enzyme catalyzing the conversion of upstream androgenic precursors to estrogens (androstenedione → estrone and testosterone → E2; **Figure 1**). In premenopausal women, estrogens are produced predominantly in the ovarian granulosa cells and are released into the bloodstream where they act primarily in an endocrine fashion. In postmenopausal women and in men, estrogen synthesis takes place in extra-gonadal tissues (liver, heart, skin/fat tissue, and brain) where estrogens act mainly as paracrine or autocrine factors. Aromatase expression in these various sites is under the control of tissue-specific promoters regulated by different cohorts of transcription factors. Therefore, aromatase activity differs substantially in various tissues and organs in health and disease [37]. Notably, human endothelium expresses a complete aromatase-estrogen-E2 receptor system [38], and increased expression of aromatase has been reported in hPASMCs from female PAH patients and in the lungs of female rats and mice with angioproliferative PH [39]. Increased aromatase activity and plasma E2 levels seen in both men and women with advanced liver disease is associated with increased risk of portopulmonary PAH [40], and increased aromatization of androgens and elevated E2 levels have been reported in postmenopausal women and in men with PAH [34, 35]. Noteworthy, E2 stimulates aromatase activity and by increasing aromatization of androgen precursors may augment its own production as well as production of E1. Because of the importance of this enzyme in estrogen synthesis, blocking aromatase activity is an important pharmacological tool used for the treatment of estrogen-dependent diseases (breast cancer, endometriosis, and endometrial cancer). Anastrozole (a third-generation aromatase inhibitor) reduces E2 levels and attenuates PH in female mice exposed to hypoxia [39] and in Sugene 5416 + hypoxia rats with angioproliferative PH [39, 41]. Moreover, when combined with the selective estrogen receptor degrader fulvestrant, anastrozole reverses PH in BMPR2-mutant mice [42]. Likewise, in PAH patients treatment with anastrozole reduces elevated E2 levels by 40% and E1 levels by 70% and significantly increases functional capacity, i.e., 6-minute-walk distance [43]. Notably, E2 augments gonadal aromatase activity, and by increasing aromatization of androgens, E2 may augment its own production as well as that of other estrogens [44]. Inflammation and inflammatory cytokines upregulate aromatase activity, and TNFα is one of the most potent inducers of aromatase. In contrast to estrogens that do not have effect on TNFα induction of aromatase [45], 2ME inhibits both basal and TNFα-stimulated aromatase activity [45–47].

In addition to aromatase, another potential source of increased estrogen production in PAH is the "sulfatase pathway." In addition to DHEA-S, other substrates for STS are biologically inactive estrone sulfate (E1-S) and estradiol sulfate (E2-S), and sulfatase plays a key role in intracrine regeneration of biologically active E2 and E1 (**Figure 1**). Inflammatory cytokines increase STS activity. More importantly, STS expression is stimulated by estrogens via estrogen receptor alpha (ERα) signaling, and at least in breast cancer, STS is upregulated by the elevated local E2 levels [26]. Thereby, in an inflammatory environment, E2 through feed-forward mechanisms may increase its on production via both the sulfatase and aromatase pathways (**Figure 2**), as implicated by elevated aromatase activity and E2 levels in both experimental PH [39] and in men and women with PAH [34, 35, 40].

2.2 Dysregulated estradiol metabolism in PAH

Once formed, E2 is primarily metabolized by oxidation at C2, C4, and C16 positions and converted to metabolites with different estrogenic activities and diverse (often opposite) biological effects. In humans, E2 hydroxylation is mediated by

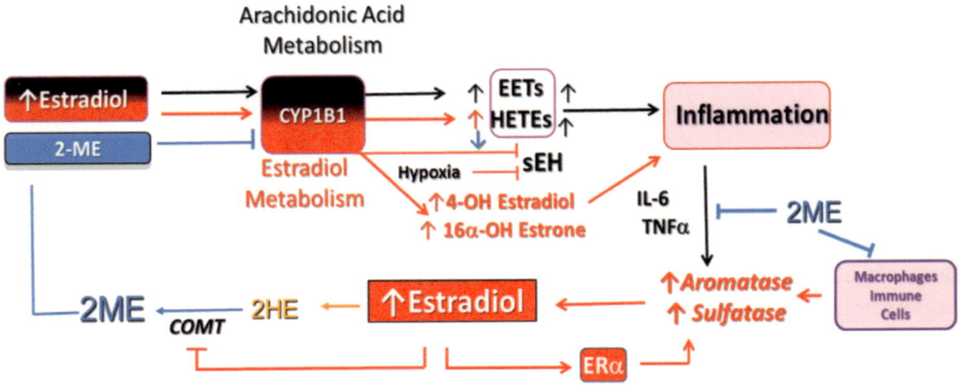

Figure 2.
Opposing effects of E2 and 2ME on estrogens and arachidonic acid metabolism. Inflammation and dual metabolic activity of CYP1B1 instigate estradiol feed-forward mechanisms that involve sulfatase, aromatase, COMT, and CYP1B1 (red arrows). Thereby, the increased E2 and arachidonic acid pro-inflammatory metabolites may contribute to the development of inflammatory and angioproliferative phenotypes in women. In contrast, 2ME by inhibiting CYP1B1 activity, macrophage influx/activation, and pro-inflammatory cytokine induction of estrogen-producing enzymes (blue arrows) balances inflammation and E2 production and its metabolisms into mitogenic pro-inflammatory and angiogenic metabolites. CYP1B1 activation results in production of pro-inflammatory arachidonic acid metabolites (black arrows). COMT = catechol-O-methyltransferase; CYP = cytochrome p450 enzymes; EETs = epoxyeicosatrienoic acids; HETEs = hydroxyeicosatetraenoic acids; sEH = soluble epoxide hydrolase, degrades EETs.

multiplying CYP450 enzymes (CYP1A1/1A2/3A4/1B1) with 2-hydroxyestradiol (2HE) being the main metabolite; however, 4-hydroxyestradiol (4HE; **Figures 1** and **2**) is formed to a lesser degree (~5%). This is followed by methylation of hydroxyl groups catalyzed by catechol-O-methyl transferase (COMT). The hydroxylation/methylation pathway is a major metabolic pathway that accounts for ~50% of E2 metabolism. It largely takes place in the liver and leads to production of 2ME, a major non-estrogenic metabolite with antiproliferative, anti-angiogenic, and anti-inflammatory effects [48]. In addition to hepatocytes and numerous cancer cell lines, conversion of E2 to downstream 2HE and 2ME takes place in cardiovascular and renal compartments [48], and a solid line of evidence suggests that 2ME mediates the antiproliferative effects of E2 in cardiovascular and renal cells [49].

Notably, the protective effects of E2 in experimental PH are mediated, at least in part, by 2ME [50, 51]. Furthermore, it seems that in highly proliferative states, 2ME may oppose estrogen-driven proliferation. For example, in highly proliferative human leiomyoma cells (hLCs) characterized by doubled ERα signaling (inherently regulated by microtubule dynamics) [52], COMT overexpression or treatment with 2ME stabilizes microtubules, attenuates E2-induced proliferation, inhibits ERα signaling, and reduces HIF-1α and aromatase expression in hLCs [53, 54]. Unfortunately, it seems that elevated E2 levels seen in PAH may adversely affect both hepatic and extrahepatic 2ME production. In this regard, men have higher COMT activity than women [55, 56], and sex hormones regulate COMT activity that is highly expressed in human and rat lungs [57, 58]. The exposure to E2 reduces hepatic COMT activity in rats [59, 60]; in vitro E2 decreases COMT transcription, activity, and protein levels [61, 62]; and tamoxifen, by antagonizing E2, increases COMT activity in peripheral tissues [63]. Together, these findings suggest that reduced COMT activity by elevated E2 and subsequent decreased in 2ME production may render women more susceptible to the development of PAH. At present it is unknown whether there is reduced 2ME production in PAH. Yet, reduced 2ME production has been linked to the development of preeclampsia [64], increased sensitivity to angiotensin II [65], and insulin resistance [66].

2.3 Opposing effects of estradiol and 2-methoxyestradiol on CYP1B1 activity and estrogen and arachidonic acid metabolism

E2 and 2ME have opposing effects on CYP1B1, another E2 metabolizing enzyme implicated in pathogenesis of PAH. Human CYP1B1 mRNA and protein are constitutively expressed in the lung and in VSMCs and ECs [67]. CYP1B1 may facilitate E2 oxidation at C4 and C16, thus producing highly estrogenic and reactive metabolites 4-hydroxyestradiol (4HE) and 16α-hydroxyestrone (16αHE1). Experimental and human data suggest a major pathogenic role for CYP1B1 and 16αHE1 in PAH. In this regard, CYP1B1 increases the risk of PAH and RV dysfunction in humans and plays a pathogenic role in the 16αHE1-BMPR2 interaction in experimental PH [68–76]. Notably, E2 and 2ME have divergent effects on CYP1B1 activity. Estradiol is not only a substrate for CYP1B1, but also it is transcriptional activator of CYP1B1 [77]. In contrast, in vitro 2ME exerts feedback inhibition on CYP1B1 activity [78]. Moreover, 2ME inhibits aryl hydrocarbon receptor-mediated induction of CYP1B1 and reduces CYP1B1 production of reactive metabolites. In vivo, 2ME significantly inhibits CYP1B1 expression and attenuates pressure overload-induced cardiac remodeling [78, 79]. In vivo CYP1B1 inhibition by 2ME reduces biosynthesis of mid-chain hydroxyeicosatetraenoic acids (HETEs) [79], suggesting a significant role for CYP1B1 in arachidonic acid metabolism. Indeed, due to its lipoxygenase-like activity, CYP1B1 facilitates arachidonic acid metabolism into HETEs and epoxyeicosatrienoic acids (EETs) [80]. In the pulmonary vasculature, EETs and HETEs have vasoconstrictive, inflammatory, and mitogenic/angiogenic effects and have been implicated in the development of experimental hypoxic PH [81–84]. Noteworthy, in PAH patients increased production of HETEs correlates with a poor prognosis [85]. E2 not only stimulates production of HETEs and EETs but also by inhibiting expression/activity of soluble epoxide hydrolase (sEH) [86] suppresses the degradation of EETs. Several lines of evidence link low sEH activity to the pathophysiology of PH: (1) the lungs from PH patients express no/little sEH; (2) E2-, genetic-, and pharmacologically induced downregulation of sEH potentiates hypoxic vasoconstriction; (3) hypoxia downregulates sEH; and (3) sEH−/− mice have exacerbated pulmonary vascular remodeling when exposed to chronic hypoxia [87–89]. Therefore, elevated E2 levels in PAH through a feed-forward mechanism may shift both E2 and AA metabolism toward production of pro-inflammatory/angiogenic/mitogenic metabolites. Based on its inhibitory effects, 2ME should suppress the production of these pathogenic E2 and AA metabolites (**Figure 2**).

3. Divergent effects of 2ME and estradiol in pulmonary endothelium in PAH

Dysregulated angiogenesis with formation of occlusive and plexiform lesions is a hallmark of PAH. Although estrogens provide protection in healthy systemic vascular beds, they have opposite effects on malignant proangiogenic/highly proliferative vessels [90] that share many similarities with vascular changes in PAH. The highly proliferative apoptosis-resistant cells in the central core of vascular lesions in PAH have elevated MAPK activity; increased expression of HIF-1α, VEGF protein, and VEGF-2 receptor; and low expression of p27kip1 (marker of low cell growth) [15, 16]. In human pulmonary artery ECs (hPAECs) and at physiological concentrations (1–10 nM), E2 (1) stimulates cell proliferation [91]; (2) promotes the phosphorylation of p42/44 and p38 MAPK via ERs; (3) downregulates the cell cycle inhibitor p27Kip1; (4) stimulates cell migration; (5) induces HIF-1α expression and VEGF synthesis; and (6) protects against apoptosis [92–94]. Also, E2 stimulates proliferation of human pulmonary artery vascular smooth muscle cells (hPASMCs). In canine pulmonary arterial segments, E2 tends to inhibit proliferation of PASMCs in segments with intact endothelium but significantly enhances proliferation in segments stripped of endothelium [95], suggesting opposite effects of E2 in intact versus injured pulmonary vessels. Thereby, in the pulmonary vasculature exposed to known and unknown multiple hits, estrogens may potentiate pathological endothelial remodeling in PAH (**Figure 3**).

In contrast to E2, it is well established that 2ME has strong anti-angiogenic, antiproliferative, and pro-apoptotic effects [96] and thereby may prevent PAH or inhibit the progression of PAH. In this regard, of particular importance for PAH are the effects of 2ME on the HIF-1α/VEGF axis. One of the most consistently reported effects of 2ME is HIF-1α downregulation, and 2ME has been increasingly used as pharmacological tool to inhibit HIF-1α in numerous studies outside the PAH field. HIF-1α transcriptional activity regulates more than 40 genes and respective proteins, including those that play a key role in vascular reactivity and angiogenesis [97, 98]. The role of HIF-1α in PAH is supported by multiple findings including the following: (1) obliterative endothelial lesions in severe PH in humans overexpress HIF-1α [15]; (2) in experimental PH there is similar increase in HIF-1α that correlates with the development of PH and pulmonary vascular remodeling and RV hypertrophy; (3) heterozygous deficiency in HIF-1α protects against the development of PH [99, 100]; and (4) pathologic normoxic HIF-1α signaling activation leads to the glycolytic shift (the Warburg effect) in highly proliferative ECs [101].

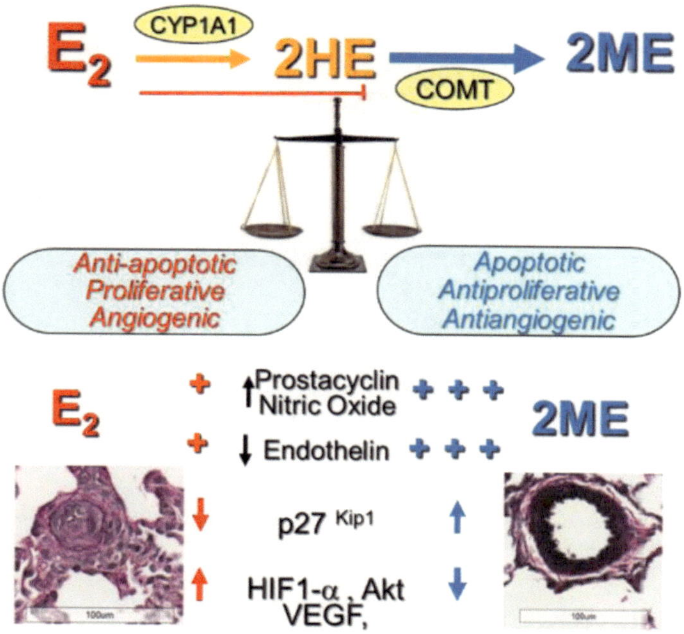

Figure 3.
In the injured highly proliferative/angiogenic endothelium in pulmonary vasculature in PAH, 2ME behaves as biological antagonist of estradiol (E2). 2ME and E2 have opposite effects on key regulators of angioproliferation (p27Kip1, AKT, HIF1-α, VEGF), and 2ME is a more potent modulator of prostacyclin, endothelin, and nitric oxide synthesis/release than E2.

Hypoxia stimulates 2ME formation which inhibits the production of hypoxia-driven angiogenesis and angiogenic cytokines (VEGF and FGF-2) [31, 102]. Therefore, 2ME should be viewed as a local modulator that fine-tunes the rate of angiogenesis. Recent studies in experimental PH support the notion of 2ME as a local anti-angiogenic factor in PAH and E2 as promoter of angiogenesis. For example, (1) basal HIF-1α protein expression is higher in female hPASMCs than in males; (2) the antimitogenic effects of 2ME in hPASMCs are associated with reduced HIF-1α expression; (3) 2ME attenuates intermittent and chronic hypoxia-induced PH [22, 103, 104]; (4) in both male and female hypoxic PH rats, 2ME attenuates the disease while decreasing HIF-1α protein expression [103]; (5) female rats with Sugene 5416 + hypoxia (SU+Hx)-induced PH have more severe occlusive and plexiform lesions and sporadically develop grade 6 lesions (necrotizing arteritis); (6) E2 exacerbates angioproliferative lesions and perivascular inflammation in ovariectomized SU+Hx rats [105, 106]; and (7) in intact female SU+Hx rats, 2ME, but not E2, exhibits therapeutic effects [107]. The effects of 2ME in PAH patients are unknown. Yet, at least in experimental angioproliferative PH, 2ME could be viewed as biological antagonist of E2 in the endothelium and as a modifier of "dysregulated angiogenesis."

4. Metabolic reprograming and 2ME in PAH

The major metabolic changes that take place in PAH occur in the form of the shift from oxidative phosphorylation to glycolysis. Known as the Warburg effect, this event is frequently observed and has been systematically investigated in cancer tissue. Notably, the Warburg effect has also been reported in pulmonary vasculature cells in PAH patients [108] and linked to highly proliferative, angiogenic, and apoptosis-resistant cancer cells and vascular cells in PAH. Not surprisingly, the

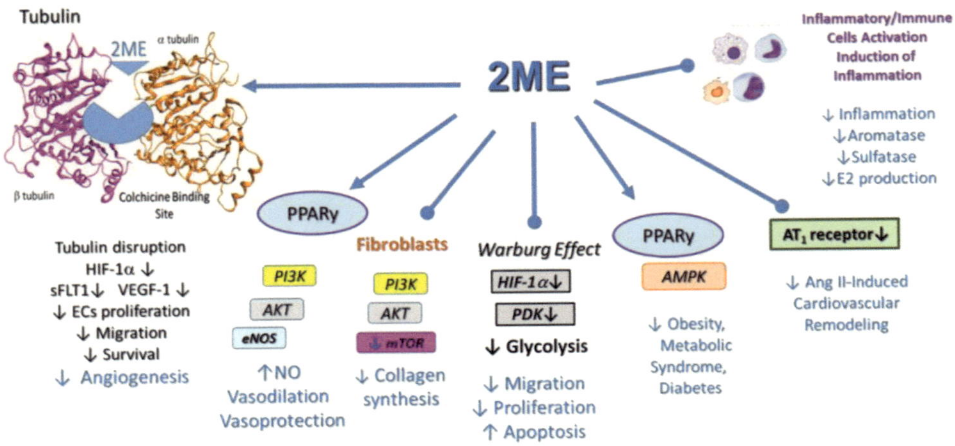

Figure 4.
Cellular effects of 2ME that contributes to the reduced E2 production, inflammation, angioproliferation, metabolic reprograming, and vascular and right ventricular remodeling in PAH.

Warburg effect has been explored as a potential anti-angiogenic target in cancer and more recently in PAH. The HIF-1α transcription factor has been identified as a master hypoxic regulator responsible for the metabolic shift in PAH [101, 109]. Hypoxic induction of HIF-1α leads to overexpression of pyruvate dehydrogenase kinase (PDK) which results in inhibition of pyruvate dehydrogenase that shunts pyruvate into glycolysis and induces conversion of glucose to lactate [108]. Dichloroacetate (DCA), a PDK inhibitor, reverses the Warburg effect and exhibits therapeutic effects in several animal models of PH [110–112]. Because 2ME is a strong HIF-1α inhibitor, 2ME should induce metabolic reprograming in PAH. Presently, the effects of 2ME on metabolic reprograming in PAH are unknown. However, 2ME inhibits lactate-induced mitochondrial biogenesis in highly proliferative osteosarcoma cells, and in apoptosis-resistant melanoma cells, 2ME attenuates proliferation and glycolysis by inhibiting HIF-1α and PDK expression [113–115]. Therefore, 2ME could be viewed as modulator of metabolic reprograming. Further studies are warranted to investigate the effects of 2ME on the Warburg effect that in PAH is associated with highly proliferative, angiogenic, and apoptosis-resistant phenotypes (**Figure 4**).

5. Anti-inflammatory and immunomodulatory effects of 2ME

Inflammation and altered immunity, i.e., perivascular accumulation of inflammatory and immune cells in pulmonary circulation, have been increasingly recognized as pathogenic factors in PAH [17–19]. In this regard, at young age women have more robust immune responses than men. Although initially beneficial, with aging these aggressive immune responses may become detrimental [116]. This may explain why various immune diseases are remarkably more frequent in women and why many immune diseases, such as systemic sclerosis (SSc), lupus, and mixed connective tissue disease, are associated with increased risk of PAH [117]. Furthermore, recently distinct immune phenotypes have been reported in PAH patients [118]. In experimental PH, dysregulated immunity in the form of deficient regulatory T-cell (Treg) activity contributes to increased inflammation [20]. Both alveolar macrophages and immune cells express steroidogenic enzymes including sulfatase and aromatase [119–121]. Inflammatory cytokines, prostanoids, and growth factors regulate the expression and activity of steroidogenic enzymes, and in turn, sex hormones may influence the production and release of these autocrine/paracrine mediators [122]. E2 upregulates CYP1B1, aromatase, and sulfatase activity and inhibits sEH activity. Therefore, in an inflammatory environment, E2 may boost its own production, and via a feed-forward mechanism, E2 may enhance the production of pro-inflammatory, angiogenic, and mitogenic estrogens and increase the accumulation of pro-inflammatory arachidonic acid metabolites (**Figure 2**). In contrast to E2, non-estrogenic 2ME exhibits significant anti-inflammatory effects, largely through suppression of tissue recruitment and activation of macrophages [123, 124]. This is one of the most consistent in vivo effects of 2ME seen in experimental models of cardiovascular and renal injury [125, 126] and in pulmonary hypertension [50, 51, 127–129]. 2ME, its metabolic precursor 2HE, and the synthetic analog 2-ethoxyestradiol inhibit influx and activation of macrophages in MCT- and bleomycin-induced PH, and this inhibition correlates with reduced PH, vascular remodeling, and fibrosis. 2ME and its metabolic precursor 2HE also inhibit the synthesis of leukotrienes [130]. Blocking of leukotriene production by macrophages prevents endothelial injury and reverses experimental PH [131]. In experimental autoimmune rheumatoid arthritis, 2ME slows down disease progression by inhibiting inflammatory cytokine mRNA (IL-1β, TNF-α, IL-6, and IL-17), leucocyte infiltration, and neovascularization [31]. In several models of autoimmune inflammatory disease, the beneficial effects of 2ME were ascribed to the inhibition of immune cell activation, proliferation, and pro-inflammatory cytokine release [31, 132–134]. Finally, in fibroblasts from SSc disease patients that are at high risk for developing PAH, 2ME reduces hypoxia-induced production of connective tissue growth factor and collagen I by inhibiting the PI3K/Akt/mTOR or HIFα signaling [135]. Collectively, these data in inflammatory and autoimmune diseases point toward 2ME as potential modulator of inflammation and immunity relevant to the development and progression of PAH.

6. 2-Methoxyestradiol and the renin-angiotensin system (RAS) in PAH

Evidence suggests that the renin-angiotensin system (RAS) contributes to the development of PAH [136, 137]. For example, (1) there is increased systemic RAS activity in patients with idiopathic PAH; (2) in experimental and human PH, ACE activity and expression are increased in PAECs, PVSMCs, plexiform lesions, and the RV; (3) increased Ang II type 1 receptor expression and signaling correlates with PAH progression and vascular remodeling [137–142]; and (4) inhibition of RAS slows down the progression of MCT-induced PH [143]. Cumulating data also suggests that 2ME may behave as biological antagonist of Ang II. 2ME downregulates Ang II type I receptors [144–146]. In COMT−/− mice that have reduced 2ME production, 2ME treatment abolishes hypersensitivity to and injury induced by Ang II [65]. Furthermore, in Cyp1B1−/− mice that also have reduced 2ME production, 2ME treatment abolishes Ang II-induced oxidative and vascular injury [147]. Finally, of relevance in PAH, in vivo in high RAS activity models, 2ME attenuates Ang II-induced cardiac and vascular remodeling and fibrosis and isoproterenol-induced RV and LV hypertrophy and fibrosis [148].

7. Role of 2ME and the metabolic syndrome in PAH

The metabolic syndrome (MS) is recognized as risk factor for PH [149, 150]. Deficiency in PPARγ (a downstream target of BMPR2) and deficiency in apolipoprotein E and adiponectin (downstream targets of PPARγ) have been linked to the development of PH in rodents [151–153]. Moreover, COMT, via methoxyestradiols, has been identified as a major factor modulating insulin resistance. The low-activity COMT158Val-Met is linked to MS [154], whereas high-activity COMT rs4680 is associated with lower HbA1c levels and protection from type 2 diabetes [155]. COMT deficiency in mice leads to disrupted glucose homeostasis [66], and 2ME which shares structural similarity with PPARγ ligands and acts as a PPARγ agonist [65, 156] (**Figure 4**) induces AMPK phosphorylation and improves insulin sensitivity in COMT−/− mice [66]. 2HE, a metabolic precursor of 2ME and COMT substrate, activates AMPK in human skeletal muscle, attenuates experimental PH in lean rats, and reduces MS-induced endothelial dysfunction in obese rats. Moreover, in rats with polygenic obesity and MS, in both PH-free females and PH male ZDSD rats, treatment with 2HE reduces glycosylated hemoglobin, RVPSP, and RV-EDP and attenuates vascular remodeling in male PH rats [157]. These data warrant further investigation of 2ME in MS-induced PH and support the notion of 2ME as potential disease modifier in MS-related PH.

8. 2-Methoxyestradiol and current pharmacotherapy of PAH

Despite significant advances in pharmacotherapy of PAH, mortality of patients with PAH remains high. Therefore, there is still a significant unmet medical need for more effective therapies. Currently approved drugs for treatment of PAH include medications that correct for prostanoid deficiency (prostanoids and prostacyclin receptor agonists) and deficiency of nitric oxide (PDE5 inhibitors and soluble guanylate cyclase stimulators) or combat overproduction of endothelin (endothelin receptor antagonists). Compared to ECs in healthy vessels, the ECs in affected vessels in PH show reduced prostacyclin and nitric oxide synthesis and overexpression of ET-1 [158–160]. Noteworthy, compared to estradiol, 2ME is a more potent inhibitor of endothelin synthesis in endothelial cells [48, 161], and 2ME and its metabolic precursor 2HE inhibit endothelin-induced vasoconstriction [162]. Furthermore, in ECs 2ME is a more potent stimulator of prostacyclin synthesis than estradiol [163, 164]. 2ME also increases basal and potentiates stimulated NO production in male and OVX female rats, but has no effect in intact females, and in vitro these effects are abolished by the eNOS inhibitor L-NAME [165]. 2ME induces vasodilation by stimulating NO release via PPARγ/PI3K/Akt pathway [166] and increases NO production in uterine artery ECs from pregnant sheep [167]. Moreover, in L-NAME-treated rats, 2ME attenuates severe hypertension and renal, cardiac, and vascular injury and inflammation and reduces mortality by 87% [125]. Likewise, 2ME exhibits beneficial effects in MCT-induced PH and efficacy comparable to that of bosentan and sildenafil. Importantly, in combination with bosentan or sildenafil, 2ME has synergistic therapeutic effects (further reduces vascular remodeling, inflammatory responses, and survival) [128]. Finally, none of the approved therapies for PAH affects endothelial remodeling and "dysregulated angiogenesis" in pulmonary vasculature; in contrast, as discussed above in Section 3, 2ME is a strong anti-angiogenic agent and inhibitor of HIF-VEGF axis that is critical for the metabolic shift and development of occlusive and complex vascular lesions. Altogether, these data clearly indicate 2ME as a promising pharmacological agent capable of providing additional benefit in PAH patients on standard single or combination therapy.

9. Pharmacokinetic aspects of the development of 2ME as a disease modifier in PAH

The safety and efficacy of 2ME in human PAH are unknown. However, over the past two decades, numerous phase I and II clinical trials have been conducted to test the safety and antitumor efficacy of 2ME in patients with solid malignancies. These studies show that 2ME is well tolerated and safe in doses up to 3 g/day. Unfortunately, even high oral doses of 2ME achieve only low plasma 2ME concentrations due to high pre-systemic metabolism (glucuronidation) in the liver. In experimental PH, therapeutic effects of 2ME are achieved by much lower doses (240 μg/kg/day) delivered by subcutaneous micro-infusions that produce high physiological concentrations of 2ME (~3 ng/ml; equivalent to levels observed during the last trimester of pregnancy) [168]. At these concentrations, 2ME does not induce estrogenic effects. In rats with MCT-induced PH, although higher doses of 2ME do not additionally reduce PH and RV hypertrophy, higher doses do further inhibit media remodeling and inflammation [127]. Likewise, in contrast to oral administration in healthy volunteers and cancer patients, subcutaneous administration of a long-acting formulation of 2ME in doses up to 10 mg produced blood levels of 2ME >1 ng/ml over a 3-week period, with no estrogenic or other adverse effects reported [169]. Currently, various parenteral formulations of 2ME with supposedly high bioavailability are under investigation.

10. Conclusions and future directions

An expanding body of knowledge indicates that many of the beneficial cellular and systemic effects of E2 are due, at least in part, to its major and non-estrogenic metabolite 2ME. This underscores the importance of estradiol metabolism to 2ME in women's health and suggests that 2ME deficiency may contribute to many female predominant diseases, including PAH. 2ME should not be viewed only as partial mediator of E2 effects but in PAH should be considered a moderator of the harmful effects of estrogens related to several key events in PAH including altered estradiol and arachidonic acid metabolism, angiogenesis, inflammation, harmful immune responses, metabolic syndrome, and metabolic reprograming. The above discussion hopefully makes the case for 2ME as unrecognized disease modifier in PAH.

Conflict of interest

The authors do not have any conflict of interest.

Author details

Stevan P. Tofovic[1,2,3*] and Edwin K. Jackson[2]

1 Heart, Lung, Blood and Vascular Medicine Institute, University of Pittsburgh School of Medicine, Pittsburgh, Pennsylvania, USA

2 Department of Pharmacology and Chemical Biology, University of Pittsburgh School of Medicine, Pittsburgh, Pennsylvania, USA

3 Department of Medicine, University of Pittsburgh School of Medicine, Pittsburgh, Pennsylvania, USA

*Address all correspondence to: tofovic@pitt.edu

References

[1] Dresdale DT, Schultz M, Michtom RJ. Primary pulmonary hypertension. I. Clinical and hemodynamic study. American Journal of Medicine. 1951;**11**:686-705

[2] Wood P. Pulmonary hypertension. British Medical Bulletin. 1952;**8**:348-353

[3] Benza RL, Miller DP, Barst RJ, Badesch DB, Frost AE, McGoon MD. An evaluation of long-term survival from time of diagnosis in pulmonary arterial hypertension from the REVEAL registry. Chest. 2012;**142**:448-456. DOI: 10.1378/chest.11-1460

[4] Benza RL, Miller DP, Gomberg-Maitland M, Frantz RP, Foreman AJ, Coffey CS, et al. Predicting survival in pulmonary arterial hypertension: Insights from the registry to evaluate early and long-term pulmonary arterial hypertension disease management (REVEAL). Circulation. 2010;**122**:164-172. DOI: 10.1161/CIRCULATIONAHA.109.898122

[5] Escribano-Subias P, Blanco I, Lopez-Meseguer M, Lopez-Guarch CJ, Roman A, Morales P, et al. Survival in pulmonary hypertension in Spain: Insights from the spanish registry. The European Respiratory Journal. 2012;**40**:596-603. DOI: 10.1183/09031936.00101211

[6] Humbert M, Sitbon O, Chaouat A, Bertocchi M, Habib G, Gressin V, et al. Survival in patients with idiopathic, familial, and anorexigen-associated pulmonary arterial hypertension in the modern management era. Circulation. 2010;**122**:156-163. DOI: 10.1161/CIRCULATIONAHA.109.911818

[7] Humbert M, Sitbon O, Yaici A, Montani D, O'Callaghan DS, Jais X, et al. Survival in incident and prevalent cohorts of patients with pulmonary arterial hypertension. The European Respiratory Journal. 2010;**36**:549-555. DOI: 10.1183/09031936.00057010

[8] Jing ZC, Xu XQ, Han ZY, Wu Y, Deng KW, Wang H, et al. Registry and survival study in Chinese patients with idiopathic and familial pulmonary arterial hypertension. Chest. 2007;**132**:373-379. DOI: 10.1378/chest.06-2913

[9] Tamura Y, Kumamaru H, Satoh T, Miyata H, Ogawa A, Tanabe N, et al. Effectiveness and outcome of pulmonary arterial hypertension-specific therapy in Japanese patients with pulmonary arterial hypertension. Circulation Journal: Official Journal of the Japanese Circulation Society. 2017;**82**:275-282. DOI: 10 1253/circj.CJ-17-0139

[10] Humbert M, Sitbon O, Chaouat A, Bertocchi M, Habib G, Gressin V, et al. Pulmonary arterial hypertension in France: Results from a national registry. American Journal of Respiratory and Critical Care Medicine. 2006;**173**:1023-1030. DOI: 10.1164/rccm.200510-1668OC

[11] McGoon MD, Miller DP. REVEAL: A contemporary US pulmonary arterial hypertension registry. European Respiratory Review: An Official Journal of the European Respiratory Society. 2012;**21**:8-18. DOI: 10.1183/09059180.00008211

[12] Zhang R, Dai LZ, Xie WP, Yu ZX, Wu BX, Pan L, et al. Survival of Chinese patients with pulmonary arterial hypertension in the modern treatment era. Chest. 2011;**140**:301-309. DOI: 10.1378/chest.10-2327

[13] Hoeper MM, Huscher D, Ghofrani HA, Delcroix M, Distler O, Schweiger C, et al. Elderly patients diagnosed with idiopathic pulmonary arterial hypertension: Results from the

COMPERA registry. International Journal of Cardiology. 2013;**168**:871-880. DOI: 10.1016/j.ijcard.2012.10.026

[14] Pietra GG, Capron F, Stewart S, Leone O, Humbert M, Robbins IM, et al. Pathologic assessment of vasculopathies in pulmonary hypertension. Journal of the American College of Cardiology. 2004;**43**:25S-32S. DOI: 10.1016/j.jacc.2004.02.033

[15] Cool CD, Stewart JS, Werahera P, Miller GJ, Williams RL, Voelkel NF, et al. Three-dimensional reconstruction of pulmonary arteries in plexiform pulmonary hypertension using cell-specific markers. Evidence for a dynamic and heterogeneous process of pulmonary endothelial cell growth. The American Journal of Pathology. 1999;**155**:411-419. DOI: 10.1016/S0002-9440(10)65137-1

[16] Tuder RM, Chacon M, Alger L, Wang J, Taraseviciene-Stewart L, Kasahara Y, et al. Expression of angiogenesis-related molecules in plexiform lesions in severe pulmonary hypertension: Evidence for a process of disordered angiogenesis. The Journal of Pathology. 2001;**195**:367-374. DOI: 10.1002/path.953

[17] Hassoun PM, Mouthon L, Barbera JA, Eddahibi S, Flores SC, Grimminger F, et al. Inflammation, growth factors, and pulmonary vascular remodeling. Journal of the American College of Cardiology. 2009;**54**:S10-S19. DOI: 10.1016/j.jacc.2009.04.006

[18] Kuebler WM, Bonnet S, Tabuchi A. Inflammation and autoimmunity in pulmonary hypertension: Is there a role for endothelial adhesion molecules? (2017 Grover conference series). Pulmonary Circulation. 2018;**8**:2045893218757596. DOI: 10.1177/2045893218757596

[19] Rabinovitch M, Guignabert C, Humbert M, Nicolls MR. Inflammation and immunity in the pathogenesis of pulmonary arterial hypertension. Circulation Research. 2014;**115**:165-175. DOI: 10.1161/CIRCRESAHA.113.301141

[20] Tamosiuniene R, Tian W, Dhillon G, Wang L, Sung YK, Gera L, et al. Regulatory T cells limit vascular endothelial injury and prevent pulmonary hypertension. Circulation Research. 2011;**109**:867-879. DOI: 10.1161/CIRCRESAHA.110.236927

[21] Stacher E, Graham BB, Hunt JM, Gandjeva A, Groshong SD, McLaughlin VV, et al. Modern age pathology of pulmonary arterial hypertension. American Journal of Respiratory and Critical Care Medicine. 2012;**186**:261-272. DOI: 10.1164/rccm.201201-0164OC

[22] Tofovic SP, Zhang X, Jones T, Jackson EK, Petrusevska G. 2-Methoxyestradiol attenuates the development and retards the progression of chronic hypoxia-induced pulmonary hypertension in rats. Circulation. 2005;**112**:98-99

[23] Mikkaichi T, Suzuki T, Tanemoto M, Ito S, Abe T. The organic anion transporter (OATP) family. Drug Metabolism and Pharmacokinetics. 2004;**19**:171-179

[24] Obaidat A, Roth M, Hagenbuch B. The expression and function of organic anion transporting polypeptides in normal tissues and in cancer. Annual Review of Pharmacology and Toxicology. 2012;**52**:135-151. DOI: 10.1146/annurev-pharmtox-010510-100556

[25] Radford DJ, Wang K, McNelis JC, Taylor AE, Hechenberger G, Hofmann J, et al. Dehydroepiandrosterone sulfate directly activates protein kinase C-beta to increase human neutrophil superoxide generation. Molecular Endocrinology. 2010;**24**:813-821. DOI: 10.1210/me.2009-0390

[26] Mueller JW, Gilligan LC, Idkowiak J, Arlt W, Foster PA. The regulation of steroid action by sulfation and desulfation. Endocrine Reviews. 2015;**36**:526-563. DOI: 10.1210/er.2015-1036

[27] Bonnet S, Dumas-de-La-Roque E, Begueret H, Marthan R, Fayon M, Dos Santos P, et al. Dehydroepiandrosterone (DHEA) prevents and reverses chronic hypoxic pulmonary hypertension. Proceedings of the National Academy of Sciences of the United States of America. 2003;**100**:9488-9493. DOI: 10.1073/pnas.1633724100

[28] Dumas de la Roque E, Quignard JF, Ducret T, Dahan D, Courtois A, Begueret H, et al. Beneficial effect of dehydroepiandrosterone on pulmonary hypertension in a rodent model of pulmonary hypertension in infants. Pediatric Research. 2013;**74**:163-169. DOI: 10.1038/pr.2013.73

[29] Hampl V, Bibova J, Povysilova V, Herget J. Dehydroepiandrosterone sulphate reduces chronic hypoxic pulmonary hypertension in rats. The European Respiratory Journal. 2003;**21**:862-865

[30] Oka M, Karoor V, Homma N, Nagaoka T, Sakao E, Golembeski SM, et al. Dehydroepiandrosterone upregulates soluble guanylate cyclase and inhibits hypoxic pulmonary hypertension. Cardiovascular Research. 2007;**74**:377-387. DOI: 10.1016/j.cardiores.2007.01.021

[31] Plum SM, Park EJ, Strawn SJ, Moore EG, Sidor CF, Fogler WE. Disease modifying and antiangiogenic activity of 2-methoxyestradiol in a murine model of rheumatoid arthritis. BMC Musculoskeletal Disorders. 2009;**10**:46. DOI: 10.1186/1471-2474-10-46

[32] Alzoubi A, Toba M, Abe K, O'Neill KD, Rocic P, Fagan KA, et al. Dehydroepiandrosterone restores right ventricular structure and function in rats with severe pulmonary arterial hypertension. American Journal of Physiology Heart and Circulatory Physiology. 2013;**304**:H1708-H1718. DOI: 10.1152/ajpheart.00746.2012

[33] Homma N, Nagaoka T, Karoor V, Imamura M, Taraseviciene-Stewart L, Walker LA, et al. Involvement of RhoA/Rho kinase signaling in protection against monocrotaline-induced pulmonary hypertension in pneumonectomized rats by dehydroepiandrosterone. American Journal of Physiology Lung Cellular and Molecular Physiology. 2008;**295**:L71-L78. DOI: 10.1152/ajplung.90251.2008

[34] Baird GL, Archer-Chicko C, Barr RG, Bluemke DA, Foderaro AE, Fritz JS, et al. Lower DHEA-S levels predict disease and worse outcomes in post-menopausal women with idiopathic, connective tissue disease- and congenital heart disease-associated pulmonary arterial hypertension. The European Respiratory Journal. 2018;**51**(6). DOI: 10.1183/13993003.00467-2018

[35] Ventetuolo CE, Baird GL, Barr RG, Bluemke DA, Fritz JS, Hill NS, et al. Higher estradiol and lower dehydroepiandrosterone-sulfate levels are associated with pulmonary arterial hypertension in men. American Journal of Respiratory and Critical Care Medicine. 2016;**193**:1168-1175. DOI: 10.1164/rccm.201509-1785OC

[36] Dumas de La Roque E, Savineau JP, Metivier AC, Billes MA, Kraemer JP, Doutreleau S, et al. Dehydroepiandrosterone (DHEA) improves pulmonary hypertension in chronic obstructive pulmonary disease (COPD): A pilot study. Annales D'endocrinologie. 2012;**73**:20-25. DOI: 10.1016/j.ando.2011.12.005

[37] Simpson ER, Zhao Y, Agarwal VR, Michael MD, Bulun SE, Hinshelwood

MM, et al. Aromatase expression in health and disease. Recent Progress in Hormone Research. 1997;**52**:185-213 discussion 213-4

[38] Simpson ER, Clyne C, Rubin G, Boon WC, Robertson K, Britt K, et al. Aromatase—A brief overview. Annual Review of Physiology. 2002;**64**:93-127. DOI: 10.1146/annurev.physiol.64.081601.142703

[39] Mair KM, Wright AF, Duggan N, Rowlands DJ, Hussey MJ, Roberts S, et al. Sex-dependent influence of endogenous estrogen in pulmonary hypertension. American Journal of Respiratory and Critical Care Medicine. 2014;**190**:456-467. DOI: 10.1164/rccm.201403-0483OC

[40] Roberts KE, Fallon MB, Krowka MJ, Brown RS, Trotter JF, Peter I, et al. Genetic risk factors for portopulmonary hypertension in patients with advanced liver disease. American Journal of Respiratory and Critical Care Medicine. 2009;**179**:835-842. DOI: 10.1164/rccm.200809-1472OC

[41] Tofovic S, Bilan V, Mi Z, Jackson EK, Schneider F. Aromatase inhibition attenuates and ovariectomy and 4-hydroxyestradiol have mixed effects on development of angioproliferative pulmonary hypertension in female rats. American Journal of Respiratory and Critical Care Medicine. 2013;**187**:A6099

[42] Chen X, Austin ED, Talati M, Fessel JP, Farber-Eger EH, Brittain EL, et al. Oestrogen inhibition reverses pulmonary arterial hypertension and associated metabolic defects. The European Respiratory Journal. 2017;**50**. DOI: 10.1183/13993003.02337-2016

[43] Kawut SM, Archer-Chicko CL, DeMichele A, Fritz JS, Klinger JR, Ky B, et al. Anastrozole in pulmonary arterial hypertension. A randomized, double-blind, placebo-controlled trial. American Journal of Respiratory and Critical Care Medicine. 2017;**195**:360-368. DOI: 10.1164/rccm.201605-1024OC

[44] Adashi EY, Hsueh AJ. Estrogens augment the stimulation of ovarian aromatase activity by follicle-stimulating hormone in cultured rat granulosa cells. The Journal of Biological Chemistry. 1982;**257**:6077-6083

[45] Schmidt M, Hartung R, Capellino S, Cutolo M, Pfeifer-Leeg A, Straub RH. Estrone/17beta-estradiol conversion to, and tumor necrosis factor inhibition by, estrogen metabolites in synovial cells of patients with rheumatoid arthritis and patients with osteoarthritis. Arthritis and Rheumatism. 2009;**60**:2913-2922. DOI: 10.1002/art.24859

[46] Capellino S, Straub RH, Cutolo M. Aromatase and regulation of the estrogen-to-androgen ratio in synovial tissue inflammation: Common pathway in both sexes. Annals of the New York Academy of Sciences. 2014;**1317**:24-31. DOI: 10.1111/nyas.12398

[47] Purohit A, Singh A, Ghilchik MW, Reed MJ. Inhibition of tumor necrosis factor alpha-stimulated aromatase activity by microtubule-stabilizing agents, paclitaxel and 2-methoxyestradiol. Biochemical and Biophysical Research Communications. 1999;**261**:214-217. DOI: 10.1006/bbrc.1999.1010

[48] Dubey RK, Tofovic SP, Jackson EK. Cardiovascular pharmacology of estradiol metabolites. The Journal of Pharmacology and Experimental Therapeutics. 2004;**308**:403-409. DOI: 10.1124/jpet.103.058057

[49] Dubey RK, Imthurn B, Jackson EK. 2-methoxyestradiol: A potential treatment for multiple proliferative disorders. Endocrinology. 2007;**148**:4125-4127. DOI: 10.1210/en.2007-0514

[50] Tofovic SP, Zhang X, Jackson EK, Dacic S, Petrusevska G.

2-methoxyestradiol mediates the protective effects of estradiol in monocrotaline-induced pulmonary hypertension. Vascular Pharmacology. 2006;**45**:358-367. DOI: 10.1016/j.vph.2006.05.007

[51] Tofovic SP, Zhang X, Jackson EK, Zhu H, Petrusevska G. 2-methoxyestradiol attenuates bleomycin-induced pulmonary hypertension and fibrosis in estrogen-deficient rats. Vascular Pharmacology. 2009;**51**:190-197. DOI: 10.1016/j.vph.2009.06.002

[52] Manavathi B, Acconcia F, Rayala SK, Kumar R. An inherent role of microtubule network in the action of nuclear receptor. Proceedings of the National Academy of Sciences of the United States of America. 2006;**103**:15981-15986. DOI: 10.1073/pnas.0607445103

[53] Salama SA, Kamel MW, Botting S, Salih SM, Borahay MA, Hamed AA, et al. Catechol-o-methyltransferase expression and 2-methoxyestradiol affect microtubule dynamics and modify steroid receptor signaling in leiomyoma cells. PLoS One. 2009;**4**:e7356. DOI: 10.1371/journal.pone.0007356

[54] Salama SA, Nasr AB, Dubey RK, Al-Hendy A. Estrogen metabolite 2-methoxyestradiol induces apoptosis and inhibits cell proliferation and collagen production in rat and human leiomyoma cells: A potential medicinal treatment for uterine fibroids. Journal of the Society for Gynecologic Investigation. 2006;**13**:542-550. DOI: 10.1016/j.jsgi.2006.09.003

[55] Boudikova B, Szumlanski C, Maidak B, Weinshilboum R. Human liver catechol-O-methyltransferase pharmacogenetics. Clinical Pharmacology and Therapeutics. 1990;**48**:381-389

[56] Floderus Y, Ross SB, Wetterberg L. Erythrocyte catechol-O-methyltransferase activity in a swedish population. Clinical Genetics. 1981;**19**:389-392

[57] Bryan-Lluka LJ. Evidence for saturation of catechol-O-methyltransferase by low concentrations of noradrenaline in perfused lungs of rats. Naunyn-Schmiedeberg's Archives of Pharmacology. 1995;**351**:408-416

[58] De Santi C, Giulianotti PC, Pietrabissa A, Mosca F, Pacifici GM. Catechol-O-methyltransferase: Variation in enzyme activity and inhibition by entacapone and tolcapone. European Journal of Clinical Pharmacology. 1998;**54**:215-219

[59] Cohn CK, Axelrod J. The effect of estradiol on catechol-O-methyltransferase activity in rat liver. Life Sciences Pt. 1: Physiology and Pharmacology. 1971;**10**:1351-1354

[60] Parvez S, Parvez SH, Youdim MB. Variation in activity of monoamine metabolizing enzymes in rat liver during pregnancy. British Journal of Pharmacology. 1975;**53**:241-246

[61] Jiang H, Xie T, Ramsden DB, Ho SL. Human catechol-O-methyltransferase down-regulation by estradiol. Neuropharmacology. 2003;**45**:1011-1018

[62] Xie T, Ho SL, Ramsden D. Characterization and implications of estrogenic down-regulation of human catechol-O-methyltransferase gene transcription. Molecular Pharmacology. 1999;**56**:31-38

[63] Schendzielorz N, Rysa A, Reenila I, Raasmaja A, Mannisto PT. Complex estrogenic regulation of catechol-O-methyltransferase (COMT) in rats. Journal of Physiology and Pharmacology: An Official Journal

of the Polish Physiological Society. 2011;**62**:483-490

[64] Wantania J, Attamimi A, Siswishanto R. A comparison of 2-methoxyestradiol value in women with severe preeclampsia versus normotensive pregnancy. Journal of Clinical and Diagnostic Research: JCDR. 2017;**11**:QC35-QC38. DOI: 10.7860/JCDR/2017/21516.9603

[65] Ueki N, Kanasaki K, Kanasaki M, Takeda S, Koya D. Catechol-O-methyltransferase deficiency leads to hypersensitivity of the pressor response against angiotensin II. Hypertension. 2017;**69**:1156-1164. DOI: 10.1161/HYPERTENSIONAHA.117.09247

[66] Kanasaki M, Srivastava SP, Yang F, Xu L, Kudoh S, Kitada M, et al. Deficiency in catechol-o-methyltransferase is linked to a disruption of glucose homeostasis in mice. Scientific Reports. 2017;7:7927. DOI: 10.1038/s41598-017-08513-w

[67] Kerzee JK, Ramos KS. Constitutive and inducible expression of Cyp1a1 and Cyp1b1 in vascular smooth muscle cells: Role of the Ahr bHLH/PAS transcription factor. Circulation Research. 2001;**89**:573-582

[68] Austin ED, Cogan JD, West JD, Hedges LK, Hamid R, Dawson EP, et al. Alterations in oestrogen metabolism: Implications for higher penetrance of familial pulmonary arterial hypertension in females. The European Respiratory Journal. 2009;**34**:1093-1099. DOI: 10.1183/09031936.00010409

[69] Chen X, Talati M, Fessel JP, Hemnes AR, Gladson S, French J, et al. Estrogen metabolite 16alpha-hydroxyestrone exacerbates bone morphogenetic protein receptor type II-associated pulmonary arterial hypertension through MicroRNA-29-mediated modulation of cellular metabolism. Circulation. 2016;**133**:82-97. DOI: 10.1161/CIRCULATIONAHA.115.016133

[70] Hood KY, Montezano AC, Harvey AP, Nilsen M, MacLean MR, Touyz RM. Nicotinamide adenine dinucleotide phosphate oxidase-mediated redox signaling and vascular remodeling by 16alpha-hydroxyestrone in human pulmonary artery cells: Implications in pulmonary arterial hypertension. Hypertension. 2016;**68**:796-808. DOI: 10.1161/HYPERTENSIONAHA.116.07668

[71] Johansen AK, Dean A, Morecroft I, Hood K, Nilsen M, Loughlin L, et al. The serotonin transporter promotes a pathological estrogen metabolic pathway in pulmonary hypertension via cytochrome P450 1B1. Pulmonary Circulation. 2016;**6**:82-92. DOI: 10.1086/685023

[72] Loyd JE. Pulmonary arterial hypertension: Insights from genetic studies. Proceedings of the American Thoracic Society. 2011;**8**:154-157. DOI: 10.1513/pats.201007-047MS

[73] Ventetuolo CE, Mitra N, Wan F, Manichaikul A, Barr RG, Johnson C, et al. Oestradiol metabolism and androgen receptor genotypes are associated with right ventricular function. The European Respiratory Journal. 2016;**47**:553-563. DOI: 10.1183/13993003.01083-2015

[74] Ventetuolo CE, Ouyang P, Bluemke DA, Tandri H, Barr RG, Bagiella E, et al. Sex hormones are associated with right ventricular structure and function: The MESA-right ventricle study. American Journal of Respiratory and Critical Care Medicine. 2011;**183**:659-667. DOI: 10.1164/rccm.201007-1027OC

[75] West J, Cogan J, Geraci M, Robinson L, Newman J, Phillips JA, et al. Gene expression in BMPR2 mutation carriers with and without evidence of pulmonary arterial hypertension suggests pathways relevant to disease penetrance. BMC Medical Genomics. 2008;**1**:45. DOI: 10.1186/1755-8794-1-45

[76] White K, Johansen AK, Nilsen M, Ciuclan L, Wallace E, Paton L, et al. Activity of the estrogen-metabolizing enzyme cytochrome P450 1B1 influences the development of pulmonary arterial hypertension. Circulation. 2012;**126**:1087-1098. DOI: 10.1161/CIRCULATIONAHA.111.062927

[77] Tsuchiya Y, Nakajima M, Yokoi T. Cytochrome P450-mediated metabolism of estrogens and its regulation in human. Cancer Letters. 2005;**227**:115-124. DOI: 10.1016/j.canlet.2004.10.007

[78] Dawling S, Roodi N, Parl FF. Methoxyestrogens exert feedback inhibition on cytochrome P450 1A1 and 1B1. Cancer Research. 2003;**63**:3127-3132

[79] Maayah ZH, Levasseur J, Siva Piragasam R, Abdelhamid G, Dyck JRB, Fahlman RP, et al. 2-methoxyestradiol protects against pressure overload-induced left ventricular hypertrophy. Scientific Reports. 2018;**8**:2780. DOI: 10.1038/s41598-018-20613-9

[80] Choudhary D, Jansson I, Stoilov I, Sarfarazi M, Schenkman JB. Metabolism of retinoids and arachidonic acid by human and mouse cytochrome P450 1b1. Drug Metabolism and Disposition: The Biological Fate of Chemicals. 2004;**32**:840-847

[81] Jiang J, Wang S, Wang Z, Ma J, Liu S, Li W, et al. The role of ERK1/2 in 15-HETE-inhibited apoptosis in pulmonary arterial smooth muscle cells. Journal of Receptor and Signal Transduction Research. 2011;**31**:45-52. DOI: 10.3109/10799893.2010.512013

[82] Ma C, Li Y, Ma J, Liu Y, Li Q, Niu S, et al. Key role of 15-lipoxygenase/15-hydroxyeicosatetraenoic acid in pulmonary vascular remodeling and vascular angiogenesis associated with hypoxic pulmonary hypertension. Hypertension. 2011;**58**:679-688. DOI: 10.1161/HYPERTENSIONAHA.111.171561

[83] Maayah ZH, Althurwi HN, Abdelhamid G, Lesyk G, Jurasz P, El-Kadi AO. CYP1B1 inhibition attenuates doxorubicin-induced cardiotoxicity through a mid-chain HETEs-dependent mechanism. Pharmacological Research. 2016;**105**:28-43. DOI: 10.1016/j.phrs.2015.12.016

[84] Sugumaran PK, Wang S, Song S, Nie X, Zhang L, Feng Y, et al. 15-oxo-eicosatetraenoic acid prevents serum deprivation-induced apoptosis of pulmonary arterial smooth muscle cells by activating pro-survival pathway. Prostaglandins, Leukotrienes, and Essential Fatty Acids. 2014;**90**:89-98. DOI: 10.1016/j.plefa.2014.01.006

[85] Al-Naamani N, Sagliani KD, Dolnikowski GG, Warburton RR, Toksoz D, Kayyali U, et al. Plasma 12- and 15-hydroxyeicosanoids are predictors of survival in pulmonary arterial hypertension. Pulmonary Circulation. 2016;**6**:224-233. DOI: 10.1086/686311

[86] Yang YM, Sun D, Kandhi S, Froogh G, Zhuge J, Huang W, et al. Estrogen-dependent epigenetic regulation of soluble epoxide hydrolase via DNA methylation. Proceedings of the National Academy of Sciences of the United States of America. 2018;**115**:613-618. DOI: 10.1073/pnas.1716016115

[87] Kandhi S, Qin J, Froogh G, Jiang H, Luo M, Wolin MS, et al. EET-dependent potentiation of pulmonary arterial pressure: Sex-different regulation of soluble epoxide hydrolase. American Journal of Physiology Lung Cellular and Molecular Physiology. 2015;**309**:L1478-L1486. DOI: 10.1152/ajplung.00208.2015

[88] Kandhi S, Zhang B, Froogh G, Qin J, Alruwaili N, Le Y, et al. EETs promote hypoxic pulmonary vasoconstriction via constrictor prostanoids. American Journal of Physiology Lung Cellular and Molecular Physiology.

2017;**313**:L350-L359. DOI: 10.1152/ajplung.00038.2017

[89] Keseru B, Barbosa-Sicard E, Schermuly RT, Tanaka H, Hammock BD, Weissmann N, et al. Hypoxia-induced pulmonary hypertension: Comparison of soluble epoxide hydrolase deletion vs. inhibition. Cardiovascular Research. 2010;**85**: 232-240. DOI: 10.1093/cvr/cvp281

[90] Klouche M. Estrogens in human vascular diseases. Annals of the New York Academy of Sciences. 2006;**1089**:431-443. DOI: 10.1196/annals.1386.032

[91] Lippert C, Seeger H, Mueck AO, Lippert TH. The effects of A-ring and D-ring metabolites of estradiol on the proliferation of vascular endothelial cells. Life Sciences. 2000;**67**:1653-1658

[92] Geraldes P, Sirois MG, Bernatchez PN, Tanguay JF. Estrogen regulation of endothelial and smooth muscle cell migration and proliferation: Role of p38 and p42/44 mitogen-activated protein kinase. Arteriosclerosis, Thrombosis, and Vascular Biology. 2002;**22**:1585-1590

[93] Spyridopoulos I, Sullivan AB, Kearney M, Isner JM, Losordo DW. Estrogen-receptor-mediated inhibition of human endothelial cell apoptosis. Estradiol as a survival factor. Circulation. 1997;**95**:1505-1514

[94] Suzuma I, Mandai M, Takagi H, Suzuma K, Otani A, Oh H, et al. 17 beta-estradiol increases VEGF receptor-2 and promotes DNA synthesis in retinal microvascular endothelial cells. Investigative Ophthalmology & Visual Science. 1999;**40**:2122-2129

[95] Farhat MY, Vargas R, Dingaan B, Ramwell PW. In vitro effect of oestradiol on thymidine uptake in pulmonary vascular smooth muscle cell: Role of the endothelium. British Journal of Pharmacology. 1992;**107**:679-683

[96] Tofovic SP. Estrogens and development of pulmonary hypertension: Interaction of estradiol metabolism and pulmonary vascular disease. Journal of Cardiovascular Pharmacology. 2010;**56**:696-708. DOI: 10.1097/FJC.0b013e3181f9ea8d

[97] Semenza GL. HIF-1 and human disease: One highly involved factor. Genes & Development. 2000;**14**:1983-1991

[98] Semenza GL. HIF-1: Mediator of physiological and pathophysiological responses to hypoxia. Journal of Applied Physiology. 2000;**88**:1474-1480. DOI: 10.1152/jappl.2000.88.4.1474

[99] Lai YL, Law TC. Chronic hypoxia- and monocrotaline-induced elevation of hypoxia-inducible factor-1 alpha levels and pulmonary hypertension. Journal of Biomedical Science. 2004;**11**:315-321. DOI: 10.1159/000077099

[100] Liu W, Zhang Y, Lu L, Wang L, Chen M, Hu T. Expression and correlation of hypoxia-inducible factor-1alpha (HIF-1alpha) with pulmonary artery remodeling and right ventricular hypertrophy in experimental pulmonary embolism. Medical Science Monitor: International Medical Journal of Experimental and Clinical Research. 2017;**23**:2083-2088

[101] Fitzgerald G, Soro-Arnaiz I, De Bock K. The Warburg effect in endothelial cells and its potential as an anti-angiogenic target in cancer. Frontiers in Cell and Developmental Biology. 2018;**6**:100. DOI: 10.3389/fcell.2018.00100

[102] Basini G, Grasselli F, Bussolati S, Baioni L, Bianchi F, Musci M, et al. Hypoxia stimulates the production of the angiogenesis inhibitor 2-methoxyestradiol by swine granulosa cells. Steroids. 2011;**76**:1433-1436. DOI: 10.1016/j.steroids.2011.07.012

[103] Docherty CK, Nilsen M, MacLean MR. Influence of 2-methoxyestradiol and sex on hypoxia-induced pulmonary hypertension and hypoxia-inducible factor-1-alpha. Journal of the American Heart Association. 2019;**8**:e011628, 10.1161/JAHA.118.011628

[104] Hao S, Jiang L, Fu C, Wu X, Liu Z, Song J, et al. 2-methoxyestradiol attenuates chronic-intermittent-hypoxia-induced pulmonary hypertension through regulating microRNA-223. Journal of Cellular Physiology. 2019;**234**(5):6324-6335. DOI: 10.1002/jcp.27363

[105] Tofovic SPRO, Jackson EK, Champion H, Schneider F. Estrogens exacerbates development of occlusive pulmonary arterial hypertension and formation of plexiform lesions. American Journal of Respiratory and Critical Care Medicine. 2012;**185**:A6803

[106] Tofovic SP, Bilan V, Jackson EK, Schneider F. Sugene 5416 dose-hypoxia-normoxia-gender interaction in angioproliferative pulmonary hypertension in rats. American Journal of Respiratory and Critical Care Medicine. 2014;**189**:A5566

[107] Tofovic SP, Rafikova O. Preventive and therapeutic effects of 2-methoxyestradiol, but not estradiol, in severe occlusive pulmonary arterial hypertension in female rats. American Journal of Respiratory and Critical Care Medicine. 2009;**179**:A1802

[108] Chan SY, Rubin LJ. Metabolic dysfunction in pulmonary hypertension: From basic science to clinical practice. European Respiratory Review: An Official Journal of the European Respiratory Society. 2017;**26**. DOI: 10.1183/16000617.0094-2017

[109] Tuder RM, Davis LA, Graham BB. Targeting energetic metabolism: A new frontier in the pathogenesis and treatment of pulmonary hypertension. American Journal of Respiratory and Critical Care Medicine. 2012;**185**:260-266. DOI: 10.1164/rccm.201108-1536PP

[110] Li B, Yan J, Shen Y, Liu Y, Ma Z. Dichloroacetate prevents but not reverses the formation of neointimal lesions in a rat model of severe pulmonary arterial hypertension. Molecular Medicine Reports. 2014;**10**:2144-2152. DOI: 10.3892/mmr.2014.2432

[111] McMurtry MS, Bonnet S, Wu X, Dyck JR, Haromy A, Hashimoto K, et al. Dichloroacetate prevents and reverses pulmonary hypertension by inducing pulmonary artery smooth muscle cell apoptosis. Circulation Research. 2004;**95**:830-840. DOI: 10.1161/01.RES.0000145360.16770.9f

[112] Michelakis ED, McMurtry MS, Wu XC, Dyck JR, Moudgil R, Hopkins TA, et al. Dichloroacetate, a metabolic modulator, prevents and reverses chronic hypoxic pulmonary hypertension in rats: Role of increased expression and activity of voltage-gated potassium channels. Circulation. 2002;**105**:244-250

[113] Gorska-Ponikowska M, Kuban-Jankowska A, Daca A, Nussberger S. 2-methoxyestradiol reverses the pro-carcinogenic effect of L-lactate in osteosarcoma 143B cells. Cancer Genomics & Proteomics. 2017;**14**:483-493. DOI: 10.21873/cgp.20058

[114] Gorska-Ponikowska M, Kuban-Jankowska A, Eisler SA, Perricone U, Lo Bosco G, Barone G, et al. 2-methoxyestradiol affects mitochondrial biogenesis pathway and succinate dehydrogenase complex flavoprotein subunit a in osteosarcoma Cancer cells. Cancer Genomics & Proteomics. 2018;**15**:73-89. DOI: 10.21873/cgp.20067

[115] Zhao H, Jiang H, Li Z, Zhuang Y, Liu Y, Zhou S, et al. 2-methoxyestradiol

enhances radiosensitivity in radioresistant melanoma MDA-MB-435R cells by regulating glycolysis via HIF-1alpha/PDK1 axis. International Journal of Oncology. 2017;**50**:1531-1540. DOI: 10.3892/ijo.2017.3924

[116] Osman MS, Michelakis ED. Immunity comes to play in the "sex paradox" of pulmonary arterial hypertension. Circulation Research. 2018;**122**:1635-1637. DOI: 10.1161/CIRCRESAHA.118.313075

[117] Batton KA, Austin CO, Bruno KA, Burger CD, Shapiro BP, Fairweather D. Sex differences in pulmonary arterial hypertension: Role of infection and autoimmunity in the pathogenesis of disease. Biology of Sex Differences. 2018;**9**:15. DOI: 10.1186/s13293-018-0176-8

[118] Sweatt AJ, Hedlin HK, Balasubramanian V, Hsi A, Blum LK, Robinson WH, et al. Discovery of distinct immune phenotypes using machine learning in pulmonary arterial hypertension. Circulation Research. 2019;**124**:904-919. DOI: 10.1161/CIRCRESAHA.118.313911

[119] Berstein LM, Larionov AA, Poroshina TE, Zimarina TS, Leenman EE. Aromatase (CYP19) expression in tumor-infiltrating lymphocytes and blood mononuclears. Journal of Cancer Research and Clinical Oncology. 2002;**128**:173-176. DOI: 10.1007/s00432-002-0322-9

[120] Hennebold JD, Daynes RA. Regulation of macrophage dehydroepiandrosterone sulfate metabolism by inflammatory cytokines. Endocrinology. 1994;**135**:67-75. DOI: 10.1210/endo.135.1.8013393

[121] Schmidt M, Kreutz M, Loffler G, Scholmerich J, Straub RH. Conversion of dehydroepiandrosterone to downstream steroid hormones in macrophages. The Journal of Endocrinology. 2000;**164**:161-169

[122] Rubinow KB. An intracrine view of sex steroids, immunity, and metabolic regulation. Molecular Metabolism. 2018;**15**:92-103. DOI: 10.1016/j.molmet.2018.03.001

[123] Shand FH, Langenbach SY, Keenan CR, Ma SP, Wheaton BJ, Schuliga MJ, et al. In vitro and in vivo evidence for anti-inflammatory properties of 2-methoxyestradiol. The Journal of Pharmacology and Experimental Therapeutics. 2011;**336**:962-972. DOI: 10.1124/jpet.110.174854

[124] Sutherland TE, Anderson RL, Hughes RA, Altmann E, Schuliga M, Ziogas J, et al. 2-methoxyestradiol—A unique blend of activities generating a new class of anti-tumour/anti-inflammatory agents. Drug Discovery Today. 2007;**12**:577-584. DOI: 10.1016/j.drudis.2007.05.005

[125] Tofovic SP, Salah EM, Dubey RK, Melhem MF, Jackson EK. Estradiol metabolites attenuate renal and cardiovascular injury induced by chronic nitric oxide synthase inhibition. Journal of Cardiovascular Pharmacology. 2005;**46**:25-35

[126] Zhang X, Jia Y, Jackson EK, Tofovic SP. 2-methoxyestradiol and 2-ethoxyestradiol retard the progression of renal disease in aged, obese, diabetic ZSF1 rats. Journal of Cardiovascular Pharmacology. 2007;**49**:56-63. DOI: 10.1097/FJC.0b013e31802cb88e

[127] Tofovic SP, Jones T, Petrusevska G. Dose-dependent therapeutic effects of 2-methoxyestradiol on monocrotaline-induced pulmonary hypertension and vascular remodelling. Prilozi. 2010;**31**:279-295

[128] Tofovic SP, Jones T, Bilan VP, Jackson EK, Petrusevska G. Synergistic therapeutic effects of 2-methoxyestradiol with either sildenafil or bosentan on amelioration of monocrotaline-induced pulmonary

hypertension and vascular remodeling. Journal of Cardiovascular Pharmacology. 2010;**56**:475-483. DOI: 10.1097/FJC.0b013e3181f215e7

[129] Tofovic SP, Salah EM, Mady HH, Jackson EK, Melhem MF. Estradiol metabolites attenuate monocrotaline-induced pulmonary hypertension in rats. Journal of Cardiovascular Pharmacology. 2005;**46**:430-437

[130] Alanko J, Sievi E, Lahteenmaki T, Mucha I, Vapaatalo H, Parantainen J. Catechol estrogens as inhibitors of leukotriene synthesis. Biochemical Pharmacology. 1998;**55**:101-104

[131] Tian W, Jiang X, Tamosiuniene R, Sung YK, Qian J, Dhillon G, et al. Blocking macrophage leukotriene b4 prevents endothelial injury and reverses pulmonary hypertension. Science Translational Medicine. 2013;**5**:200ra117. DOI: 10.1126/scitranslmed.3006674

[132] Duncan GS, Brenner D, Tusche MW, Brustle A, Knobbe CB, Elia AJ, et al. 2-Methoxyestradiol inhibits experimental autoimmune encephalomyelitis through suppression of immune cell activation. Proceedings of the National Academy of Sciences of the United States of America. 2012;**109**:21034-21039. DOI: 10.1073/pnas.1215558110

[133] Luc JG, Paulin R, Zhao JY, Freed DH, Michelakis ED, Nagendran J. 2-Methoxyestradiol: A hormonal metabolite modulates stimulated T-cells function and proliferation. Transplantation Proceedings. 2015;**47**:2057-2066. DOI: 10.1016/j.transproceed.2015.05.021

[134] Xu L, Yang T, Su S, Wang F. 2-methoxyestradiol alleviates experimental autoimmune uveitis by inhibiting lymphocytes proliferation and T cell differentiation. BioMed Research International. 2016;**2016**:7948345. DOI: 10.1155/2016/7948345

[135] Zhou X, Liu C, Lu J, Zhu L, Li M. 2-Methoxyestradiol inhibits hypoxia-induced scleroderma fibroblast collagen synthesis by phosphatidylinositol 3-kinase/Akt/mTOR signalling. Rheumatology (Oxford, England). 2018;**57**:1675-1684. DOI: 10.1093/rheumatology/key166

[136] de Man FS, Tu L, Handoko ML, Rain S, Ruiter G, Francois C, et al. Dysregulated renin-angiotensin-aldosterone system contributes to pulmonary arterial hypertension. American Journal of Respiratory and Critical Care Medicine. 2012;**186**:780-789. DOI: 10.1164/rccm.201203-0411OC

[137] Morrell NW, Stenmark KR. The renin-angiotensin system in pulmonary hypertension. American Journal of Respiratory and Critical Care Medicine. 2013;**187**:1138-1139. DOI: 10.1164/rccm.201210-1872LE

[138] Morrell NW, Atochina EN, Morris KG, Danilov SM, Stenmark KR. Angiotensin converting enzyme expression is increased in small pulmonary arteries of rats with hypoxia-induced pulmonary hypertension. The Journal of Clinical Investigation. 1995;**96**:1823-1833. DOI: 10.1172/JCI118228

[139] Morrell NW, Danilov SM, Satyan KB, Morris KG, Stenmark KR. Right ventricular angiotensin converting enzyme activity and expression is increased during hypoxic pulmonary hypertension. Cardiovascular Research. 1997;**34**:393-403

[140] Morrell NW, Morris KG, Stenmark KR. Role of angiotensin-converting enzyme and angiotensin II in development of hypoxic pulmonary hypertension. The American Journal of Physiology. 1995;**269**:H1186-H1194. DOI: 10.1152/ajpheart.1995.269.4.H1186

[141] Morrell NW, Upton PD, Kotecha S, Huntley A, Yacoub MH, Polak JM, et al.

Angiotensin II activates MAPK and stimulates growth of human pulmonary artery smooth muscle via AT1 receptors. The American Journal of Physiology. 1999;**277**:L440-L448. DOI: 10.1152/ajplung.1999.277.3.L440

[142] Orte C, Polak JM, Haworth SG, Yacoub MH, Morrell NW. Expression of pulmonary vascular angiotensin-converting enzyme in primary and secondary plexiform pulmonary hypertension. The Journal of Pathology. 2000;**192**:379-384. DOI: 10.1002/1096-9896(2000)9999:9999<::AID-PATH715>3.0.CO;2-Q

[143] Ahn BH, Park HK, Cho HG, Lee HA, Lee YM, Yang EK, et al. Estrogen and enalapril attenuate the development of right ventricular hypertrophy induced by monocrotaline in ovariectomized rats. Journal of Korean Medical Science. 2003;**18**:641-648. DOI: 10.3346/jkms.2003.18.5.641

[144] Koganti S, Snyder R, Gumaste U, Karamyan VT, Thekkumkara T. 2-methoxyestradiol binding of GPR30 down-regulates angiotensin AT(1) receptor. European Journal of Pharmacology. 2014;**723**:131-140. DOI: 10.1016/j.ejphar.2013.10.064

[145] Koganti S, Snyder R, Thekkumkara T. Pharmacologic effects of 2-methoxyestradiol on angiotensin type 1 receptor down-regulation in rat liver epithelial and aortic smooth muscle cells. Gender Medicine. 2012;**9**:76-93. DOI: 10.1016/j.genm.2012.01.008

[146] Ogola B, Zhang Y, Iyer L, Thekkumkara T. 2-Methoxyestradiol causes matrix metalloproteinase 9-mediated transactivation of epidermal growth factor receptor and angiotensin type 1 receptor downregulation in rat aortic smooth muscle cells. American Journal of Physiology Cell Physiology. 2018;**314**:C554-C568. DOI: 10.1152/ajpcell.00152.2017

[147] Pingili AK, Davidge KN, Thirunavukkarasu S, Khan NS, Katsurada A, Majid DSA, et al. 2-methoxyestradiol reduces angiotensin II-induced hypertension and renal dysfunction in ovariectomized female and intact male mice. Hypertension. 2017;**69**:1104-1112. DOI: 10.1161/HYPERTENSIONAHA.117.09175

[148] Salah E, Bastacky SI, Jackson EK, Tofovic SP. 2-Methoxyestradiol attenuates angiotensin II-induced hypertension, cardiovascular remodeling, and renal injury. Journal of Cardiovascular Pharmacology. 2019;**73**:165-177. DOI: 10.1097/FJC.0000000000000649

[149] Assad TR, Hemnes AR. Metabolic dysfunction in pulmonary arterial hypertension. Current Hypertension Reports. 2015;**17**:20. DOI: 10.1007/s11906-014-0524-y

[150] Naderi N, Boobejame P, Bakhshandeh H, Amin A, Taghavi S, Maleki M. Insulin resistance in pulmonary arterial hypertension, is it a novel disease modifier? Research in Cardiovascular Medicine. 2014;**3**:e19710. DOI: 10.5812/cardiovascmed.19710

[151] Hansmann G, Wagner RA, Schellong S, Perez VA, Urashima T, Wang L, et al. Pulmonary arterial hypertension is linked to insulin resistance and reversed by peroxisome proliferator-activated receptor-gamma activation. Circulation. 2007;**115**:1275-1284. DOI: 10.1161/CIRCULATIONAHA.106.663120

[152] Summer R, Walsh K, Medoff BD. Obesity and pulmonary arterial hypertension: Is adiponectin the molecular link between these conditions? Pulmonary Circulation. 2011;**1**:440-447. DOI: 10.4103/2045-8932.93542

[153] Umar S, Partow-Navid R, Ruffenach G, Iorga A, Moazeni S,

Eghbali M. Severe pulmonary hypertension in aging female apolipoprotein E-deficient mice is rescued by estrogen replacement therapy. Biology of Sex Differences. 2017;**8**:9. DOI: 10.1186/s13293-017-0129-7

[154] Annerbrink K, Westberg L, Nilsson S, Rosmond R, Holm G, Eriksson E. Catechol O-methyltransferase val158-met polymorphism is associated with abdominal obesity and blood pressure in men. Metabolism: Clinical and Experimental. 2008;**57**:708-711. DOI: 10.1016/j.metabol.2008.01.012

[155] Hall KT, Jablonski KA, Chen L, Harden M, Tolkin BR, Kaptchuk TJ, et al. Catechol-O-methyltransferase association with hemoglobin A1c. Metabolism: Clinical and Experimental. 2016;**65**:961-967. DOI: 10.1016/j.metabol.2016.04.001

[156] Barchiesi F, Jackson EK, Fingerle J, Gillespie DG, Odermatt B, Dubey RK. 2-methoxyestradiol, an estradiol metabolite, inhibits neointima formation and smooth muscle cell growth via double blockade of the cell cycle. Circulation Research. 2006;**99**:266-274. DOI: 10.1161/01.RES.0000233318.85181.2e

[157] Tofovic SP, Hu J, Jackson EK. Schneider F 2-hydroxyestradiol attenuates metabolic syndrome-induced pulmonary hypertension. American Journal of Respiratory and Critical Care Medicine. 2015;**191**:A4096

[158] Giaid A, Saleh D. Reduced expression of endothelial nitric oxide synthase in the lungs of patients with pulmonary hypertension. The New England Journal of Medicine. 1995;**333**:214-221. DOI: 10.1056/NEJM199507273330403

[159] Giaid A, Yanagisawa M, Langleben D, Michel RP, Levy R, Shennib H, et al. Expression of endothelin-1 in the lungs of patients with pulmonary hypertension. The New England Journal of Medicine. 1993;**328**:1732-1739. DOI: 10.1056/NEJM199306173282402

[160] Tuder RM, Cool CD, Geraci MW, Wang J, Abman SH, Wright L, et al. Prostacyclin synthase expression is decreased in lungs from patients with severe pulmonary hypertension. American Journal of Respiratory and Critical Care Medicine. 1999;**159**:1925-1932. DOI: 10.1164/ajrccm.159.6.9804054

[161] Dubey RK, Jackson EK, Keller PJ, Imthurn B, Rosselli M. Estradiol metabolites inhibit endothelin synthesis by an estrogen receptor-independent mechanism. Hypertension. 2001;**37**:640-644

[162] Hill BJ, Gebre S, Schlicker B, Jordan R, Necessary S. Nongenomic inhibition of coronary constriction by 17ss-estradiol, 2-hydroxyestradiol, and 2-methoxyestradiol. Canadian Journal of Physiology and Pharmacology. 2010;**88**:147-152. DOI: 10.1139/Y09-120

[163] Seeger H, Mueck AO, Lippert TH. Effect of estradiol metabolites on prostacyclin synthesis in human endothelial cell cultures. Life Sciences. 1999;**65**:PL167-PL170

[164] Tsukamoto A, Kaneko Y, Yoshida T, Han K, Ichinose M, Kimura S. 2-Methoxyestradiol, an endogenous metabolite of estrogen, enhances apoptosis and beta-galactosidase expression in vascular endothelial cells. Biochemical and Biophysical Research Communications. 1998;**243**:9-12. DOI: 10.1006/bbrc.1998.8902

[165] Fenoy FJ, Hernandez ME, Hernandez M, Quesada T, Salom MG, Hernandez I. Acute effects of 2-methoxyestradiol on endothelial aortic No release in male and ovariectomized female rats. Nitric oxide:

Biology and Chemistry. 2010;**23**:12-19. DOI: 10.1016/j.niox.2010.03.002

[166] Chen W, Cui Y, Zheng S, Huang J, Li P, Simoncini T, et al. 2-methoxyestradiol induces vasodilation by stimulating NO release via PPARgamma/PI3K/Akt pathway. PLoS One. 2015;**10**:e0118902. DOI: 10.1371/journal.pone.0118902

[167] Landeros RV, Pastore MB, Magness RR. Effects of the catechol and methoxy metabolites of 17beta-estradiol on nitric oxide production by ovine uterine artery endothelial cells. Reproductive Sciences. 2019;**26**:459-468. DOI: 10.1177/1933719118783265

[168] Berg D, Sonsalla R, Kuss E. Concentrations of 2-methoxyoestrogens in human serum measured by a heterologous immunoassay with an 125I-labelled ligand. Acta Endocrinologica. 1983;**103**:282-288

[169] Tofovic SP, Jackson EK, Piche C. Pharmacokinetics and safety of a subcutaneously injected long-acting formulation of 2-methoxyestradiol (2ME) in healthy volunteers. Basic & Clinical Pharmacology & Toxicology. 2009;**105**:107